Medical Research, Audit and Teaching: the Essentials for Career Success

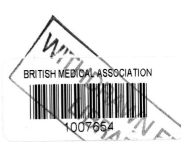

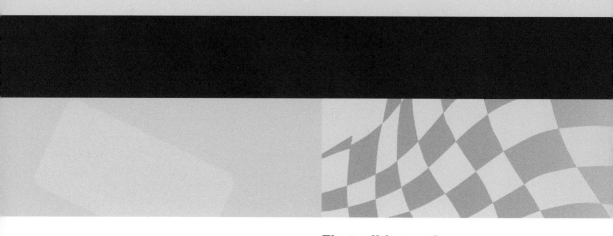

First edition author:

Amit Kaura

2nd Edition
CRASH COURSE

SERIES EDITORS

Philip Xiu
MA, MB BChir, MRCP
GP Registrar
Yorkshire Deanery
Leeds, UK

Shreelata Datta
MD, MRCOG, LLM, BSc (Hons), MBBS
Honorary Senior Lecturer
Imperial College London,
Consultant Obstetrician and Gynaecologist
King's College Hospital
London, UK

FACULTY ADVISOR

Darrel Francis
MA, MB BChir, MD, FRCP
Professor of Cardiology
Consultant Cardiologist
National Heart and Lung Institute
Hammersmith Hospital
London, UK

Medical Research, Audit and Teaching: the Essentials for Career Success

Amit Kaura
MSc(Dist), BSc(Hons), MB ChB, MRCP(UK), AFHEA, AMInstLM
Specialist Registrar in Cardiology, Imperial College Healthcare NHS Trust
NIHR Academic Clinical Fellow in Cardiology, Imperial College London
National Heart and Lung Institute
Hammersmith Hospital
London, UK

For additional online content visit StudentConsult.com

ELSEVIER

ELSEVIER

Notices

Practitioners and researchers must always rely on their own experience and knowledge in evaluating and using any information, methods, compounds or experiments described herein. Because of rapid advances in the medical sciences, in particular, independent verification of diagnoses and drug dosages should be made. To the fullest extent of the law, no responsibility is assumed by Elsevier, authors, editors or contributors for any injury and/or damage to persons or property as a matter of products liability, negligence or otherwise, or from any use or operation of any methods, products, instructions, or ideas contained in the material herein.

ISBN: 978-0-7020-7378-6
eISBN: 978-0-7020-7379-3

 your source for books, journals and multimedia in the health sciences

www.elsevierhealth.com

  Book Aid International Working together to grow libraries in developing countries

www.elsevier.com • www.bookaid.org

The publisher's policy is to use **paper manufactured from sustainable forests**

Printed in Poland
Last digit is the print number: 9 8 7 6 5 4 3 2 1

Series Editors' foreword

The *Crash Course* series was conceived by Dr Dan Horton-Szar who as series editor presided over it for more than 15 years – from publication of the first edition in 1997, until publication of the fourth edition in 2011. His inspiration, knowledge and wisdom lives on in the pages of this book. As the new series editors, we are delighted to be able to continue developing each book for the twenty-first century undergraduate curriculum.

The flame of medicine never stands still and keeping this all-new fifth series relevant for today's students is an ongoing process. Each title within this new fifth edition has been re-written to integrate basic medical science and clinical practice, after extensive deliberation and debate. We aim to build on the success of the previous titles by keeping the series up-to-date with current guidelines for best practice, and recent developments in medical research and pharmacology.

We always listen to feedback from our readers, through focus groups and student reviews of the *Crash Course* titles. For the fifth editions we have reviewed and re-written our self-assessment material to reflect today's 'single-best answer' and 'extended matching question' formats. The artwork and layout of the titles has also been largely re-worked and are now in colour, to make it easier on the eye during long sessions of revision. The new on-line materials supplement the learning process.

Despite fully revising the books with each edition, we hold fast to the principles on which we first developed the series. *Crash Course* will always bring you all the information you need to revise in compact, manageable volumes that still maintain the balance between clarity and conciseness and provide sufficient depth for those aiming at distinction. The authors are junior doctors who have recent experience of the exams you are now facing, and the accuracy of the material is checked by a team of faculty editors from across the UK.

We wish you all the best for your future careers!

Philip Xiu and Shreelata Datta

Author

Crash Course Medical Research, Audit & Teaching: the Essentials for Career Success is directed at medical students and healthcare professionals at all stages of their training. Due to the ever-growing rate at which medical knowledge is advancing, it is crucial that all professionals are able to practice and teach evidence-based medicine, which includes being able to critically appraise the medical literature. Some of the key features of this book include:

- A discussion of all **study types** using a systematic approach, therefore allowing for easy comparison.
- Essential knowledge of all commonly used **statistical methods**, using examples from real-life situations to aid understanding.
- The skills required to **critically appraise** research evidence.
- A step-by-step guide on how to get funding and **conduct your own research**.
- Knowledge on how to write high-quality abstracts and research manuscripts for **publication in high-impact factor journals**.
- Knowledge on how to get your research accepted at **local, national and international conferences**, and how to effectively present your research.
- Knowledge on how to **conduct effective audits** and quality improvement projects.
- The skills required to enhance your teaching skills and **expand your teaching portfolio**.

As with the other books in the *Crash Course* series, the material is designed to arm the reader with the essential facts on these subjects, while maintaining a balance between conciseness and clarity. References for further reading are provided where readers wish to explore a topic in greater detail.

Evidence-based medicine is a vertical theme that runs through all years of undergraduate and postgraduate study and commonly appears in exams. The self-assessment questions, which follow the modern exam format, will help the reader pass that dreaded evidence-based medicine and statistics exam with flying colours!

Not only will this book be an invaluable asset during undergraduate and postgraduate study, it will equip readers with the knowledge and skills to prepare high-quality abstracts, presentations and research manuscripts, improving their curriculum vitae in the process. This book will ensure that you have the competitive edge to excel over your colleagues in your career.

Amit Kaura

Faculty Advisor

Some people assume that clinical medicine advances by the key opinion leaders recognising the results of new research as overturning previous misconceptions and explaining to doctors as a whole why they should change their beliefs and practice.

In fact, this is not true. What happens is that key opinions leaders tend to stick to whatever they have said in the past and pretend the new research does not exist, has mysterious special flaws only recognised by them and that these new findings cannot overturn the weight of expert opinion. They very rarely say, "my previous beliefs, which I broadcast so persuasively to such great acclaim, turned out to be nonsense". Instead, they tend to reiterate their previous position, in progressively vaguer terms, and eventually retire or die. They are replaced by a new generation that have read the new research without the disadvantage of decades of incorrect assumptions, and simply accept the research findings as obvious. As the pioneering physicist Max Planck said, "science advances one funeral at a time".

The great weakness of clinical research is that unlike physical sciences, doctors are not in day-to-day practice carrying out valid scientific experiments. Instead, their exposure to science is largely limited to interpretation of science conducted by others. For this interpretation to be effective, they need to be well armed in the techniques of clinical research.

Our profession needs its young professionals and its medical students to be well prepared to design, conduct and report science that overturns the incorrect beliefs of fuddy duddies like me. This book is an excellent survey of the tools for this.

Half of my medical practice is wrong. I just don't know which half. I am hoping that readers of this book will be able to take the necessary steps to set me right!

Darrel Francis

Acknowledgements

I would like to express my deep gratitude to:

- Darrel Francis, the Faculty Advisor for this project, for his valuable and constructive suggestions during the development of this book.
- all those who have supported me in my academic career to date including Jamil Mayet, Professor of Cardiology and Clinical Director for Cardiology at Imperial College Hospital NHS Healthcare Trust.
- Jeremy Bowes, Alexandra Mortimer, Barbara Simmons and the rest of the team at Elsevier, who granted me this amazing opportunity to teach and inspire the next generation of clinical academics.
- my fiancé, Rina Patel, for all her encouragement during the preparation of this book.

I dedicate this book to:

- my dad, mum, brother Vinay, fiancé Rina, sister-in-law Kavita and the rest of my family, near and far, for their encouragement, love and support.
- my grandad and late grandmother for their unconditional support and never-ending inspiration.
- my extended family, the Patels and Singhs, for putting up with me!

Amit Kaura

Series Editors' acknowledgements

We would like to thank the support of our colleagues who have helped in the preparation of this edition, namely the junior doctor contributors who helped write the manuscript as well as the faculty editors who check the veracity of the information.

We are extremely grateful for the support of our publisher, Elsevier, whose staffs' insight and persistence has maintained the quality that Dr Horton-Szar has set-out since the first edition. Jeremy Bowes, our commissioning editor, has been a constant support. Alex Mortimer and Barbara Simmons our development editors have managed the day-to-day work on this edition with extreme patience and unflaggable determination to meet the ever looming deadlines, and we are ever grateful for Kim Benson's contribution to the online editions and additional online supplementary materials.

Philip Xiu and Shreelata Datta

Contents

Series Editors' foreword v

Prefaces vi

Acknowledgements. viii

Series Editors' acknowledgements. ix

Section 1 The essentials for career success 1

1 **An introduction to research, audit and teaching** **3**
  Book purpose 3
  Research methodology 3
  Audit and its loop 3
  Teaching theory and practice. 4
  The essentials for career success. 4
  Further reading. 4

2 **Evidence-based medicine** **5**
  What is evidence-based medicine?. 5
  Formulating clinical questions 5
  Identifying relevant evidence 6
  The search strategy 6
  Search terms. 7
  Reviewing the search strategy 7
  Critically appraising the evidence 9
  Evaluating performance .10
  Creating guideline recommendations 10
  Further reading. 11

3 **How to get involved** **13**
  Opportunities for research 13
  Types of projects. 14
  Identifying the gap in the evidence 15
  Finding a research supervisor/research group 16
  Project funding. 16
  Advice for someone considering a career in academic medicine 17
  Further reading. 18

4 **Presenting your research findings** **19**
  Submitting an abstract for presentation 19
  Selecting the right conference 19
  Writing an abstract. 20
  Poster presentations 22
  Oral presentations. 24
  Answering audience questions 27
  Further reading. 28

5 **Publishing your findings**. **29**
  Writing up a research study manuscript 29
  Submitting a manuscript for publication. 32
  Dealing with a rejected manuscript. 34
  Further reading. 36

6 **Writing a successful curriculum vitae**. **37**
  Is a curriculum vitae necessary?. 37
  What is a curriculum vitae?. 37
  Writing an effective curriculum vitae 37
  Style and formatting. 42
  Common mistakes 42
  Further reading. 42

Section 2 Research methodology 43

7 **Handling data** **45**
  Types of variables 45
  Types of data. 46
  Displaying the distribution of a single variable 47
  Displaying the distribution of two variables 49
  Describing the frequency distribution: central tendency ..51
  Describing the frequency distribution: variability. 53
  Theoretical distributions. .54
  Transformations 57
  Choosing the correct summary measure. 59
  Further reading. 60

8 **Investigating hypotheses** **61**
  Hypothesis testing 61
  Choosing a sample 61
  Extrapolating from sample to population. 62
  Comparing means and proportions: confidence intervals 66
  The *P*-value 69
  Statistical significance and clinical significance 69
  Statistical power 70
  References 76
  Further reading. 76

9 **Systematic review and meta-analysis**. **77**
  Why do we need systematic reviews?. 77
  Evidence synthesis 78
  Meta-analysis 78
  Presenting meta-analyses. 81
  Evaluating meta-analyses 81
  Key example of a meta-analysis 84
  Reporting a systematic review. 85
  References 88
  Further reading. 88

Contents

10 Research design **89**
Obtaining data 89
Interventional studies 90
Observational studies 90
Clinical trials 91
Bradford-Hill criteria for causation 92
Choosing the right study design 94
Further reading 96

11 Randomized controlled trials **97**
Why choose an interventional study design? 97
Parallel randomized controlled trial 97
Confounding, causality and bias 102
Interpreting the results 104
Types of randomized controlled trials 107
Key example of a randomized controlled trial 109
Reporting a randomized controlled trial 109
References 114
Further reading 114

12 Cohort studies **115**
Study design 115
Interpreting the results 116
Confounding, causality and bias 118
Advantages and disadvantages 122
Key example of a cohort study .122
References 124
Further reading 124

13 Case–control studies **125**
Study design 125
Interpreting the results 128
Case study: risk of constrictive pericarditis
after acute pericarditis 129
Confounding, causality and bias 130
Key example of a case–control study 134
References 136
Further reading 136

**14 Measures of disease occurrence and
cross-sectional studies** **137**
Measures of disease occurrence 137
Study design 140
Interpreting the results 142
Confounding, causality and bias 143
Key example of a cross-sectional study 146
References 148
Further reading 148

15 Ecological studies **149**
Study design 149
Interpreting the results 150
Sources of error in ecological studies 152
Key example of an ecological study 154
References 155
Further reading 155

16 Case report and case series **157**
Background 157
Conducting a case report 157
Conducting a case series 158
Critical appraisal of a case series 159
Key examples of case reports .159
Key example of a case series 159
References 160
Further reading 160

17 Qualitative research **161**
Study design 161
Organizing and analysing the data 163
Validity, reliability and transferability 164
Advantages and disadvantages 164
Key example of qualitative research 165
References 166
Further reading 166

18 Confounding **167**
What is confounding? 167
Assessing for potential confounding
factors 167
Controlling for confounding factors 168
Reporting and interpreting the results 170
Key example of study confounding 170
References 171
Further reading 171

19 Screening, diagnosis and prognosis **173**
Screening, diagnosis and prognosis 173
Screening tests 173
Example of a screening test using likelihood ratios . . . 177
Diagnostic tests 177
Evaluating the performance of a diagnostic test 178
The diagnostic process 180
Example of a diagnostic test using predictive values 184
Bias in diagnostic studies 186
Prognostic tests 187
References 190
Further reading 190

20 Statistical techniques **191**
Choosing appropriate statistical tests 191
Comparison of one group to a hypothetical value 193
Comparison of two groups 193
Comparison of three or more groups 195
Measures of association 195
Further reading 197

21 Economic evaluation **199**
What is health economics? 199
Economic question and study design 200
Cost-minimization analysis 201
Cost-utility analysis 202
Cost-effectiveness analysis 208

Cost–benefit analysis 210
Sensitivity analysis 210
Further reading 214

22 **Critical appraisal checklists** **215**
Critical appraisal 215
Critical appraisal checklist: systematic reviews
    and meta-analyses 217
Critical appraisal checklist: randomized
    controlled trials 218
Critical appraisal checklist: diagnostic studies 218
Critical appraisal checklist: qualitative studies 219
Further reading 220

23 **Crash course in statistical formulae** **221**
Describing the frequency distribution 221
Extrapolating from 'sample' to 'population' 221
Study analysis 221
Test performance 223
Economic evaluation 224
Further reading 224

**Section 3 Audit and its loop: the modern
approach to improving healthcare
practice** **225**

24 **Clinical audit** **227**
An introduction to clinical audit 227
Planning the audit 228
Choosing the standards 229
Audit protocol 229
Defining the sample 230
Data collection 230
Analysing the data 231
Evaluating the findings 231
Implementing change 232
Example of a clinical audit 232
Further reading 234

25 **Quality improvement** **235**
Quality improvement versus audit 235
The model for quality improvement 235
The aim statement 236
Measures for improvement 236
Developing the changes 237
The plan-do-study-act cycle 237
Repeating the cycle 238
Example of a quality improvement project 238
Further reading 243

**Section 4 Teaching Theory and
Practice** **245**

26 **Medical education** **247**
Introduction 247
Learning perspectives/theories 247
Optimizing learning 251
Further reading 252

27 **Designing a teaching session and teaching
    programme** **253**
Effective teaching session design 253
Setting objectives 253
Setting up a teaching programme 256
Further reading 257

28 **Teaching methods** **259**
Teaching small groups 259
Teaching in the clinical environment 261
Teaching large groups/lecturing 263
Further reading 265

29 **Teaching materials** **267**
The purpose of teaching materials 267
Different types of teaching materials 267
Social media 268
Factors influencing the type of teaching material
    to use 268
Creating effective teaching materials 268
Further reading 269

30 **Evaluation, assessment and feedback** **271**
Evaluation 271
Assessment 272
Feedback 275
References 277
Further reading 277

31 **Dealing with the student in difficulty** **279**
Recognition 279
Consultation 279
Interventions and follow-up 280
Further reading 280

Self-Assessment **281**
Single best answer (SBA) questions **283**
Extended-matching questions (EMQs) **293**
SBA answers **301**
EMQ answers **309**
Glossary **317**
Index **321**

THE ESSENTIALS FOR CAREER SUCCESS

Chapter 1

An introduction to research, audit
and teaching 3

Chapter 2

Evidence-based medicine 5

Chapter 3

How to get involved 13

Chapter 4

Presenting your research findings 19

Chapter 5

Publishing your findings 29

Chapter 6

Writing a successful curriculum vitae 37

An introduction to research, audit and teaching

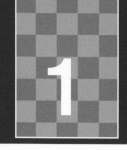

Every person who becomes a patient expects their consulting doctor to have an up-to-date working knowledge of the causes and treatment of disease in order to accurately diagnose and manage their care. All patients expect their doctor to be able to be able to weigh up the scientific evidence that is relevant to their particular condition or disease, and to recommend the best management strategy for them. In order for doctors to act in the patient's best interests, they need to be able to understand the research evidence available in their area of practice. All doctors should also be able to advise their patient on new areas of research which may be of relevance to their condition, and of active studies which may potentially question the effectiveness of current treatment strategies. Patients are also becoming a lot more knowledgeable and sophisticated and are able to appreciate that doctors who are involved in research have an aim to build on current clinical knowledge which may one day lead to improvements in the diagnosis, treatment and prevention of disease.

BOOK PURPOSE

This book aims to provide the knowledge and teach the skills to allow readers to provide high standards of patient care, achieving career success in the process. This involves having a clear understanding of essential scientific methods, principles and techniques. To achieve this, it is crucial that both undergraduate students and postgraduate doctors are equipped with the scientific skills to enable lifelong learning. The importance of acquiring these fundamental academic skills was highlighted in a report by Professor Sir Bruce Keogh. He found that hospital doctors who were more research-oriented and research-led were more likely to demonstrate high quality care. The following four sections of this book will provide you with the DNA to enable you to deliver safe and effective care to your patients:

- Research methodology
- Audit and its loop: the modern approach to improving healthcare practice
- Teaching theory and practice
- The essentials for career success

RESEARCH METHODOLOGY

Medical research encompasses 'basic science research' (also called bench science), which involves developing our understanding of more fundamental scientific principles, to clinical research, which is distinguished by the involvement of patients. The purpose of research is to discover better ways to treat and prevent disease and advance knowledge for the good of society. Undergraduate and postgraduate training are founded on established evidence through research and practice. The delivery of care to patients by healthcare professionals is based on decisions made from the best available evidence to inform diagnostic and management plans in order to meet patient needs. If there is limited evidence available in a particular area, it is the responsibility of the doctor to systematically search for it, evaluate it for scientific validity and determine whether it is applicable with respect to the decision required for the care of their patient. Every practising doctor should therefore maintain up-to-date knowledge relevant to their specialty and understand how to correctly evaluate and apply available evidence. This encompasses a key skill in being able to understand and critique statistical analyses. Overall, this forms a General Medical Council (GMC) Good Medical Practice principle, stating that doctors should 'provide effective treatments based on the best available evidence'. This principle should not be perceived as an option.

AUDIT AND ITS LOOP

Clinical audit, which is at the heart of clinical governance, involves reviewing the quality of current medical practice against explicit criteria for expected healthcare standards. Healthcare professionals should be actively involved in clinical governance to improve the quality of patient care. While clinical research aims to establish what is the best or most effective practice, clinical audit evaluates how closely local practice resembles this. Audit (and quality improvement) forms a key pillar of clinical governance, encouraging services to make better use of resources and therefore become more efficient. The data you gather during the audit process can be used to inform patients about the standard of care they are receiving. Audits may generate new research questions, which may subsequently be investigated using a

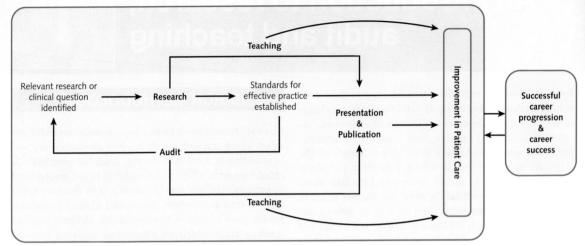

Fig. 1.1 The model for career success

research protocol. Audit and research may therefore follow each other in a continuous cycle. In an era where training doctors in management is often criticised, audits offer a good platform to learn about service provision and improvement.

TEACHING THEORY AND PRACTICE

The word 'doctor' means 'teacher' or 'learned one', and is derived from the Latin word *docere*, to teach. The GMC mandates that doctors have a professional obligation to contribute to the education and training of other doctors, medical students and nonmedical healthcare professionals on the team. Teaching activities allow you to consolidate and improve your knowledge in an area of interest, as well

as improve your communication skills, which may translate to improved interactions with patients.

THE ESSENTIALS FOR CAREER SUCCESS

Fig. 1.1 illustrates how the different sections of this book are all linked together to form a model for career success. Recruitment panels recognize the importance of research, audit, teaching and publications, with a significant number of points awarded to these activities as part of your future job applications. The skills you will acquire by the end of this book will enable you to not only provide good medical care, as defined by the GMC, but also allow you to successfully advance on the career ladder in order to reach your potential. Good luck!

● Chapter Summary

Clinical practice hones many skills that make doctors suited to research, such as teamwork, communication and analytical thinking. While not everyone should choose to pursue a long-term career in research, any time spent in research is valuable, as it will equip you with many different skills, including:

- Systematic reviewing and critical appraisal
- Numeracy (including an understanding of statistics)
- Evidence synthesis
- Communication (through teaching and publications)

FURTHER READING

British Medical Association (BMA), 2015. Every doctor a scientist and a scholar. Available from: https://www.bma.org.uk/advice/career/applying-for-a-job/every-doctor-a-scientist-and-a-scholar [Accessed 21st September 2018].

Evidence-based medicine

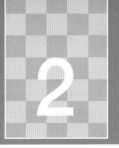

2

WHAT IS EVIDENCE-BASED MEDICINE?

Sackett and colleagues describe evidence-based medicine (a.k.a. 'evidence-based practice') as 'the conscientious, explicit and judicious use of current best evidence in making decisions about the care of individual patients'. Considering the vast rate at which medical knowledge is advancing, it is crucial for clinicians and researchers to make sense of the wealth of data (sometimes poor) that is available. Evidence-based medicine involves a number of key principles, which will be discussed in turn:

- Formulate a clinically relevant question
- Identify relevant evidence
- Systematically review and appraise the evidence identified
- Extract the most useful results and determine whether they are important in your clinical practice
- Synthesize evidence to draw conclusions
- Use the clinical research findings to generate guideline recommendations, which enable clinicians to deliver optimal clinical care to their patients
- Evaluate the implementation of evidence-based medicine

FORMULATING CLINICAL QUESTIONS

The initial step in practising evidence-based medicine involves converting a clinical encounter into a clinical question. A useful approach to formatting a clinical (or research) question is using the Patient Intervention Comparison Outcome (PICO) framework. An example is provided in Box 2.1. The question is divided in to four key components:

- *Patient/Population*: Which patients or population group of patients are you interested in? Is it necessary to consider any subgroups?

BOX 2.1   PICO MODEL

CLINICAL ENCOUNTER

John, 31 years old, was diagnosed with heart failure 3 years ago and prescribed a β-blocker which dramatically improved his symptoms. John's 5-year-old daughter, Sarah, has been recently diagnosed with chronic symptomatic congestive heart failure. John asks you, Sarah's paediatrician, whether his daughter should also be prescribed a β-blocker.
Is there a role for β-blockers in the management of heart failure in children?

Patient	Children with congestive heart failure
Intervention	Carvedilol
Comparison	No carvedilol
Outcome	Improvement of congestive heart failure symptoms

- *Intervention*: Which intervention/treatment is being evaluated?
- *Comparison/Control*: What is/are the main alternative/s compared to the intervention?
- *Outcome*: What is the most important outcome for the patient? Outcomes can include short- or long-term measures, intervention complications, social functioning or quality of life, morbidity, mortality or costs.

Not all research questions ask whether an intervention is better than existing interventions or no treatment at all. From a clinical perspective, evidence-based medicine is relevant for three other key domains:

- *Aetiology*: Is exposure to a particular agent or environment a risk factor for developing a certain condition?
- *Diagnosis*: How good is the diagnostic test (history taking, physical examination, laboratory or pathological tests and imaging) in determining whether a patient has a particular condition? Questions are usually asked about the clinical value or the diagnostic accuracy of the test (discussed in Chapter 19).

- *Prognosis*: Are there factors related to the patient that predict a particular outcome (disease progression, survival time after diagnosis of the disease, etc.)? The prognosis is based on the characteristics of the patient ('prognostic factors'; discussed in Chapter 19).

Patient experience should be taken into account when formulating the clinical question. Understandably, the *patient (P)* experience may vary depending on which patient population is being addressed. The following patient views should be determined:

- The acceptability of the proposed *i*ntervention (I) being evaluated
- Preferences for the treatment options already available (*c*omparison, C)
- What constitutes an appropriate, desired or acceptable *o*utcome (O)

Incorporating the above patient views will ensure the clinical question is patient-centred and therefore clinically relevant.

IDENTIFYING RELEVANT EVIDENCE

Sources of information

Evidence should be identified using systematic, transparent and reproducible database searches. While a number of medical databases exist, the particular source used to identify evidence of clinical effectiveness will depend on the clinical question. It is advisable that all core databases are searched for every clinical question. Depending on the subject area of the clinical question, subject-specific databases and other relevant sources should also be searched. It is important to take into account the strengths and weaknesses of each database prior to carrying out a literature search. For example, EMBASE, which is operated by Elsevier, is considered to have better coverage of European and non-English language publications and topics, such as toxicology, pharmacology, psychiatry and alternative medicine, compared to the MEDLINE database.

There is overlap between the databases; for example, there is a 10% to 87% overlap of records between EMBASE and MEDLINE. Other sources of information may include:

- Websites (e.g., ClinicalTrials.gov)
- Registries (e.g., national or regional registers)
- Conference abstracts
- Reference lists of key publications
- Personal communication with experts in the field

HINTS AND TIPS

Using 'Dr Google' to perform your entire literature search is not recommended!!!

COMMON PITFALLS

Different scientific databases cover different time periods and index different types of journals.

THE SEARCH STRATEGY

The PICO framework can be used to construct the terms for your search strategy. In other words, the framework can be used to devise the search terms for the population, which can be combined with search terms related to the intervention(s) and comparison(s) (if there are any). It is common for outcome terms to not be mentioned in the subject headings or abstracts of database records. Consequently, 'outcome' terms are often omitted from the search strategy.

SEARCH TERMS

When you input search terms, you can search for:

- a specific citation (author and publication detail)
- 'free-text' (text word) terms within the title and abstract
- subject headings with which relevant references have been tagged

Subject headings can help you identify appropriate search terms and find information on a specific topic without having to carry out further searches under all the synonyms for the preferred subject heading. For example, using the MEDLINE database, the subject heading 'heart failure' would be 'exp heart failure', where 'exp' stands for explode; i.e., the function gathers all the different subheadings within the subject heading 'heart failure'. Free-text searches are carried out to complement the subject heading searches. Free-text terms may include:

- acronyms, e.g., 'acquired immune deficiency syndrome' versus 'AIDS'
- synonyms, e.g., 'shortness of breath' versus 'breathlessness'
- abbreviations, e.g., 'echocardiography' versus 'echo'
- different spellings, e.g., 'paediatric' (UK spelling) versus 'pediatric' (US spelling).
- lay and medical terminology, e.g., 'indigestion' (lay) versus 'dyspepsia' (medical)
- brand and generic drug names, e.g., 'Septrin' (brand name) versus 'co-trimoxazole' (generic name)

It is important to identify the text word syntax (symbols) specific for each database in order to expand your results set, e.g., '.tw' used in MEDLINE. If entering two text words together, you may decide to use the term 'adj5', which indicates the two words must be adjacent within five words of each other, e.g., '(ventricular adj5 dysfunction).tw'. A symbol can be added to a word root in order to retrieve variant endings, e.g. 'smok*' or 'smok$' finds citations with the words smoked, smoker, smoke, smokes, smoking and many more. Referring to Fig. 2.1:

- in order to combine terms for the same concept (e.g., synonyms or acronyms), the Boolean operator 'OR' is used
- in order to combine sets of terms for different concepts, the Boolean operator 'AND' is used

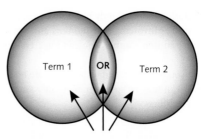

The Boolean operator 'OR' identifies all the citations that contain EITHER term

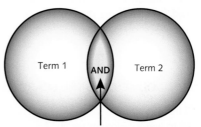

The Boolean operator 'AND' identifies all the citations that contain BOTH terms

Fig. 2.1 Boolean logic.

REVIEWING THE SEARCH STRATEGY

Expanding your results

If there are too few references following your original search, you should consider the following:

- Add symbols ($ or *) to the word root in order to retrieve variant endings
- Ensure the text word spellings are correct
- Ensure that you have combined your search terms using the correct Boolean logic concept (AND, OR)
- Consider reducing the number and type of limits applied to the search
- Ensure you have searched for related words, i.e., synonyms, acronyms
- Search for broader terms for the topic of interest

Limiting your results

If there are too many references following your original search, you should consider the following:

- Depending on the review question, you may consider limiting the search:
  - to particular study designs (e.g., searching for systematic reviews for review questions on the effectiveness of interventions)
  - by age (limiting searches by sex is not usually recommended)

COMMON PITFALLS

While subject headings are used to identify the main theme of an article, not all conditions will have a subject heading, so it is important to also search for free-text terms.

- to studies reported only in English
- to studies involving only humans and not animals
- Consider adding another Boolean logic concept (AND)
- Ensure you have searched for appropriate text words; otherwise, it may be appropriate to only search for subject headings

Documentation of the search strategy

An audit trail should be documented to ensure that the strategy used for identifying the evidence is reproducible and transparent. The following information should be documented:

- The names (and host systems) of the databases, e.g., MEDLINE (Ovid)
- The coverage dates of the database, e.g., MEDLINE (Ovid) <1946 to week 4 November 2017>
- The date on which the search was conducted
- The search strategy
- The limits that were applied to the search
- The number of records retrieved at each step of your search.

The search strategy used for the clinical question described in Box 2.1 is shown in Box 2.2 later.

BOX 2.2   DOCUMENTING THE SEARCH STRATEGY

1) MEDLINE (Ovid)
2) <1946 to week 4 November 2017>
3) Search conducted on 05/12/2017
4–6) As follows:

	History	Results
1	exp Heart Failure	115393
2	exp Ventricular Dysfunction	36190
3	cardiac failure.tw.	12080
4	heart failure.tw.	151307
5	(ventric$ adj5 dysfunction$).tw	27030
6	(ventric$ adj5 function$).tw	53518
7	1 or 2 or 3 or 4	231549
8	carvedilol.tw.	3128
9	7 and 8	1446
10	child$.tw	1304905
11	infant$.tw	385657
12	paediatr$.tw	57649
13	pediatr$.tw	259611
14	adolesc$.tw	249240
15	10 or 11 or 12 or 13 or 14	1833788
16	9 and 15	73
17	limit 9 to 'all child (0 to 18 years)'	94
18	16 or 17	108
19	limit 18 to English language	99
20	limit 19 to humans	93

CRITICALLY APPRAISING THE EVIDENCE

Once all the possible studies have been identified with the literature search, each study needs to be assessed for eligibility against objective criteria for inclusion or exclusion of studies. The studies that meet the inclusion criteria are subsequently assessed for methodological quality using a critical appraisal framework. Despite satisfying the inclusion criteria, studies appraised as being poor in quality should also be excluded.

Critical appraisal

Critical appraisal is the process of systematically examining the available evidence to judge its validity and relevance in a particular context. The appraiser should make an objective assessment of the study quality and potential for bias. It is important to determine both the internal validity and external validity of the study:

- *External validity*: The extent to which the study findings are generalisable beyond the limits of the study to the study's target population.
- *Internal validity*: Whether the study was run carefully (research design, how variables were measured, etc.) and the extent to which the observed effect(s) were produced solely by the intervention being assessed (and not by another factor).

The three main threats to internal validity (confounding, bias and causality) are discussed in turn for each of the key study designs in their respective chapters. Methodological checklists for critically appraising the key study designs covered in this book are provided in Chapter 22.

Hierarchy of evidence

Different study designs provide varying levels of evidence of causality (Fig. 2.2). The rank of a study in the hierarchy of evidence is based on its potential for bias, i.e., a systematic review provides the strongest evidence for a causal relationship between an intervention and an outcome.

> **HINTS AND TIPS**
>
> Practising medicine using unreliable evidence could lead to patient harm or limited resources being wasted – hence the importance of critical appraisal.

Assessing the results

Of the remaining studies, the reported results are extracted to a data extraction form which may include the following points:

- Does the main outcome variable measured in the study relate to the outcome variable stated in the PICO question?
- How large is the effect of interest?
- How precise is the effect of interest?/Have confidence intervals been provided? (Narrower confidence intervals indicate higher precision.)
- If the lower limit of the confidence interval represents the true value of the effect, would you consider the observed effect to be clinically significant?
- Would it be clinically significant if the upper limit of the confidence interval represented the true value of the effect?

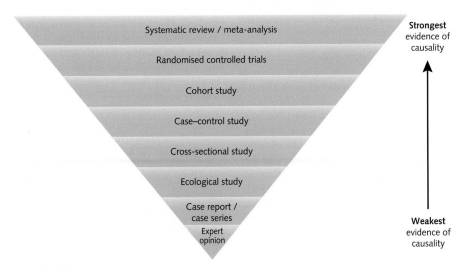

Fig. 2.2 Hierarchy of evidence.

Implementing the results

Having already critically appraised the evidence, extracted the most useful results and determined whether they are important, you must decide whether this evidence can be applied to your individual patient or population. It is important to determine whether:

- your patient has similar characteristics to those subjects enrolled in the studies from which the evidence was obtained
- the outcomes considered in the evidence are clinically important to your patient
- the study results are applicable to your patient
- the evidence regarding risks is available
- the intervention is available in your healthcare setting
- an economic analysis has been performed

The evidence regarding both efficacy and risks should be discussed with the patient in order to make an informed decision about their care.

EVALUATING PERFORMANCE

Having implemented the key evidence-based medicine principles discussed above, it is important to:

- integrate the evidence into clinical practice
- audit your performance to determine whether this approach is improving patient care (discussed in Chapter 24)
- evaluate your approach at regular intervals to determine whether there is scope for improvement in any stage of the process

CREATING GUIDELINE RECOMMENDATIONS

The evidence-based medicine approach is used to develop clinical practice guidelines. Clinical guidelines are recommendations based on the best available evidence. They are developed taking into account the views of those affected by the recommendations in the guideline, i.e., healthcare professionals, patients, their families and carers, National Health Service trusts and public and government bodies. These stakeholders play an integral part in the development of a clinical guideline and are involved in all key stages (Fig. 2.3). Topics for national clinical guideline development are highlighted by the Department of Health, based on recommendations from panels considering topic selection. Local guidelines may be commissioned by a hospital or primary care trust. The commissioning body identifies the key areas which need to be covered, which are

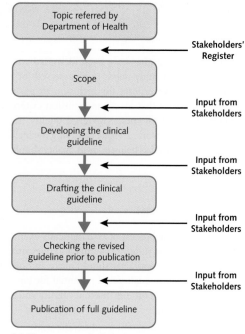

Fig. 2.3 Key stages of clinical guideline development.

subsequently translated into the scope for the clinical guideline. As highlighted by the National Institute for Health and Clinical Excellence, clinical guidelines can be used to:

- educate and train healthcare professionals
- develop standards for assessing current clinical practice
- help patients make informed decisions
- improve communication between healthcare professionals and patients

Healthcare providers and organisations should implement the recommendations with the use of slide sets, audit support and other tools tailored to need. It is important that healthcare professionals take clinical guidelines into account when making clinical decisions. However, guidelines are intended to be flexible, and clinical judgement should also be based on clinical circumstances and patient preferences.

HINTS AND TIPS

The goal of a clinical guideline is to improve the quality of clinical care delivered by healthcare professionals and to ensure that the resources used are not only efficient but also cost-effective.

Chapter Summary

- In order to practise evidence-based medicine, the initial step involves converting a clinical encounter in to a clinical question.
- A useful approach to formatting a clinical (or research) question is using the *Patient Intervention Comparison Outcome* (PICO) framework.
- Evidence should be identified using systematic, transparent and reproducible database searches.
- It is important to take into account the strengths and weaknesses of each database prior to carrying out a literature search.
- The PICO framework can be used to construct the terms for your search strategy.
- It is advisable to use subject headings and free-text terms in your search strategy.
- Once all the possible studies have been identified with the literature search, each study needs to be assessed for eligibility against objective criteria for inclusion or exclusion of studies.
- The studies that meet the inclusion criteria should subsequently be assessed for methodological quality using a critical appraisal framework.
- Critical appraisal is the process of systematically examining the available evidence to judge its validity and relevance in a particular context.
- Following critical appraisal of the evidence, you must decide whether the results can be applied to your clinical encounter.
- Clinical guidelines are recommendations based on the best available evidence.

FURTHER READING

Djulbegovic, B., Guyatt, G.H., 2017. Progress in evidence-based medicine: a quarter century on. Lancet 390 (10092), 415–423.

Lefebvre, C., Manheimer, E., Glanville, J., 2017. Chapter 6: Searching for studies. In: Higgins, J.P.T., Churchill, R., Chandler, J., Cumpston, M.S. (Eds.), Cochrane Handbook for Systematic Reviews of Interventions, Version 5.2.0 (updated February 2017), Cochrane. Available from: http://handbook-5-1.co-chrane.org [Accessed 21st September 2018].

National Institute for Health and Clinical Excellence (NICE), 2014. Developing NICE guidelines: the manual [PMG20]. Available from: https://www.nice.org.uk/guidance/pmg20/resources/developing-nice-guidelines-the-manual-pdf-72286708700869 [Accessed 21st December 2017].

Sackett, D.L., Rosenberg, W.M.C., 1995. The need for evidence based medicine. J. R. Soc. Med. 88, 620–624.

Sackett, D.L., Rosenberg, W.M.C., Gray, J.A.M., Haynes, R.B., Richardson, W.S., 1996. Evidence based medicine: What it is and what it isn't. BMJ 312, 71–72.

Straus, S., Glasziou, P., Richardson, W.S., Haynes, R.B., 2010. Evidence-Based Medicine: How to Practice and Teach It, fourth ed. Churchill-Livingstone, London.

Straus, S.E., McAlister, F.A., 2000. Evidence-based medicine: A commentary on common criticisms. CMAJ 163, 837–841.

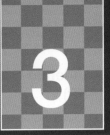

OPPORTUNITIES FOR RESEARCH

With many routes to research training available at all stages throughout your career, it is never too early, nor too late, to get involved in research and gain skills. There are plenty of opportunities to get experience in research during medical school:

- Student-selected component or module (SSC or SSM)
- Intercalated BSc degree (with potential for it to progress to a PhD)
- Collaborating with local university or hospital research groups
- Summer internship programmes

Although not essential, a track record of high academic/research performance during medical school will make you stand out more in your applications, not only for a post in the integrated academic training programme, but also for general clinical training posts. It is hard to show excellence by simply turning up to work: achievements, even small, in research allow you to prove you are interested in doing more than the bare minimum. This manifestation of initiative is something future employers will recognize as a predictor that you might show similar initiative in nonresearch activities in their department. Although first-hand research experience is recommended during both undergraduate and postgraduate training, it can also be gained through other means:

- attending journal clubs
- getting involved in smaller, ad hoc or informal research projects
- attending conferences and relevant courses (critical appraisal, research methodology, statistics, etc.)

Integrated academic training pathways

Clinical academics make up 5% to 10% of the medical workforce. In 2005, the Modernizing Medical Careers and the Joint Academic Careers Subcommittee of the UK Clinical Research Collaboration produced the Walport report, named after the chair of the Academic Careers Subcommittee, Mark Walport. The committee identified three major issues faced by academic trainees:

- Lack of flexibility in the balance of clinical and academic training and in geographical mobility.
- Lack of both a clear route of entry and a transparent career structure.
- Shortage of structured and supported posts upon completion of training.

The committee sought to resolve these three major issues and recommended the development of a clear and integrated training and career pathway for medically qualified staff to embark on a career in academic medicine. Fig. 3.1 illustrates the integrated academic training path from medical school to completion of training and beyond. While academic clinical fellowships are only available in England and Northern Ireland, the other components of the pathway are available throughout the United Kingdom. A key aspect of the training pathway is the flexibility involved in transferring between the clinical and academic training programme.

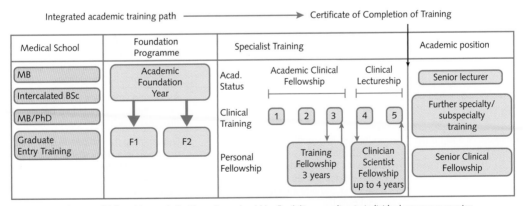

The timings of personal fellowships are indicative – there should be flexibility according to individual career progression

Fig. 3.1 The integrated academic training pathway. F1, foundation year 1 doctor; F2, foundation year 2 doctor. (Source: UK Clinical Research Collaboration, 2012. Clinical Academic Careers: England and Wales. Reproduced with permission.)

Academic Foundation Programme (AFP)

On completion of medical school, the first opportunity for research on the training pathway arises in foundation year 2. The academic attachment usually lasts for 4 months in year 2, with some ongoing academic activity during the 20 months on clinical rotation. The aim is to allow academic foundation trainees to prepare for core/speciality training or apply for an academic clinical fellowship post.

Academic clinical fellowship (ACF)

The academic clinical fellowship is intended for those who are at the start of their specialty training. The trainees are usually predoctoral clinical academics, but some appointed trainees might already have a PhD or MD. As part of the training post, which usually lasts for up to 3 years, 25% of the trainee's time is protected and devoted entirely to academic research. The aim is to allow academic clinical fellowship trainees the opportunity to identify a research interest and secure funding for a PhD or MD (training fellowship) by writing a competitive research proposal.

Academic clinical lectureship (ACL)

The academic clinical lectureship is intended for those who are postdoctoral clinical academics. As part of the training post, which usually lasts for up to 4 years, 50% of the trainee's time is dedicated entirely to postdoctoral research. The aim is to allow academic clinical lectureship trainees to progress into a senior academic role, such as a clinical scientist fellowship or a clinical senior lectureship.

TYPES OF PROJECTS

There is a wide variety of types of research and nonresearch activities that contribute to advancing medical knowledge and practice:

- Basic scientific research
- Translational research
- Clinical research
- Health services research
- Health technology research
- Epidemiological and public health studies
- Medical education research

All of these activities are valuable, and each of them plays an important role in improving patient care (Table 3.1). There are many different research methodologies, including:

- Laboratory bench work
- Systematic reviews
- Interventional studies
- Noninterventional, observational studies

Table 3.1 Types of research and nonresearch projects

Type of project	Description	Example
Basic scientific research (experimental medicine)	– Understanding pathophysiological pathways – Discovering new drug therapies	– Discovering a new cardiac biomarker
Translational research	– Translating an early stage innovation into an improvement in patient diagnosis or management	– Determining whether a newly discovered cardiac biomarker has diagnostic or prognostic value
Clinical research	– Answering clinical questions to change guidelines and clinical practice	– Comparing a novel cardiac biomarker against an established biomarker for the diagnosis of a particular cardiac disease
Health services studies	– Improving the efficiency of healthcare systems through audit and quality improvement	– Assessing whether patients with a particular cardiac disease are being managed in accordance with current best medical practice guidelines
Health technology research	– Innovating technological advances in health care	– Assessing whether a new technology-driven wearable leads to a better diagnostic yield than current technologies
Epidemiological and public health studies	– Understanding local, national and international health measures – Improving public understanding of health-related issues – Assessing and advancing health and social policies	– Determining the incidence of a medical condition in a particular population – Assessing whether a new policy has had an impact on health care access in those with low socioeconomic status
Medical education research	– Assessing and innovating the design and delivery of educational interventions	– Assessing student knowledge comparing two different teaching methods

- Economic evaluation
- Qualitative research

All research methodologies, apart from laboratory bench work, will be extensively covered in this book.

IDENTIFYING THE GAP IN THE EVIDENCE

There are no accepted standards for displaying or summarizing the gaps in knowledge, thus making it somewhat difficult for researchers, research funding bodies or guideline developers to recognize these gaps and associated research recommendations. You should discuss your interests with your supervisor or research group. They may have a project in mind if you are stuck on developing your own ideas.

Although systematic reviews (covered in Chapter 9) often provide information on what is known, they also provide useful information on what is not known.

One useful approach suggested in guideline recommendations is to apply 'level of evidence' and 'class recommendations' for all areas of management (diagnosis, treatment, prevention and rehabilitation) of a particular condition, therefore indicating whether the evidence base is insufficient (Table 3.2 and Table 3.3). Especially in those specialties in which there is an extensive research culture, such as cardiology, many obvious evidence gaps may relate to very specific comparisons or clinical outcomes within otherwise well-studied areas.

In some areas, it may be unethical, or impossible, to conduct a randomized controlled trial, in which case an observational study design may be more appropriate (please refer to Chapter 10 for a comprehensive discussion around research design). Identifying and addressing gaps in clinical evidence requires enthusiasm, dedication and collaboration between healthcare professionals. You must have a genuine interest in the research area you are entering, as you may be working on it for many months, or even years.

Developing a research question

The following questions should be considered when developing a research question:

- How important is the research question?
- Has a similar research project already been performed?
- How much value will the answer to the research question add?
- Will the research benefit patients?
- Is there already a viable solution to the question?
- What is the potential scientific and economic impact of the research being proposed?

Table 3.2 Levels of evidence

Level of evidence	Description
A	Data derived from multiple randomized clinical trials or meta-analyses
B	Data derived from a single randomized clinical trial or large nonrandomized studies
C	Consensus of opinion of the experts and/or small studies, retrospective studies, registries

Table 3.3 Classes of recommendations

Class of recommendations	Definition	Suggested wording to use
Class I	Evidence and/or general agreement that a given treatment or procedure is beneficial, useful, effective	Is recommended/is indicated
Class II	Conflicting evidence and/or a divergence of opinion about the usefulness/efficacy of the given treatment or procedure	
Class IIa	Weight of evidence/opinion is in favour of usefulness/efficacy	Should be considered
Class IIb	Usefulness/efficacy is less well established by evidence/opinion	May be considered
Class III	Evidence or general agreement that the given treatment or procedure is not useful/effective, and in some cases may be harmful	Is not recommended

- Does it align with your personal long-term career goals?
- Is a funding panel or research journal likely to find the research question of interest?

While you may be considering these questions on your own or with colleagues, most commonly you will be directed to consider a specific area by a supervisor or senior research trainee.

FINDING A RESEARCH SUPERVISOR/RESEARCH GROUP

A research project supervisor is an experienced academic who will be able to guide and support you throughout your research project from inception to publication and presentation. There are a number of key points to consider when trying to identify a research project supervisor:

- Track record – what percentage of their research projects have resulted in international presentations and high-status publications? How many trainees have they supervised?
- First-hand feedback – never join a research group without first having a confidential but frank discussion with other trainees who have previously worked with your prospective supervisor.
- Availability –how available will the prospective supervisor be? One challenge can be working for a supervisor who is a full-time clinician and has heavy clinical commitments, while your project is nonclinical in nature. At the opposite end of the spectrum, academics may spend a large proportion of their time abroad: beware of this also.
- Interests – you should get on well with and share similar research interests with your prospective supervisor.
- Working environment – is there a good research culture or vibe? What is the size of the research group, and do members all work well together? Does your project fit in with what other team members are working on? Do they collaborate with other research groups with a good reputation?

PROJECT FUNDING

Funding is available for all types of research activities, e.g., vacation research projects, research electives, intercalated research projects, PhD bursaries, research training fellowships or senior clinical research posts. With hundreds of organisations and charitable trusts that offer funding opportunities in healthcare research in the United Kingdom and thousands of opportunities worldwide, applying for funding can be confusing. All funding bodies have different eligibility criteria, application processes and deadlines. As a medical student or junior doctor, you should expect your supervisor to be able to direct you to plausible sources of funding and advise you on how to apply for it.

Before committing to an exit from clinical work in order to take on a post in full-time research, make sure that there is a sensible plan for funding. In some cases, funding has been preapplied for and obtained by the supervisor. In other cases, the supervisor is awaiting award of such funds, and you may be involved in the application process. Quite often there is a hybrid situation, with some funding already in place and hope that the rest will be received in time. It is important to ensure that the supervisor either has adequate funding for you or will support you with an application for adequate funding. Get the situation clear in your head.

Funding opportunities

The following list is of major bodies could be considered when seeking funding:

- Government funding
  - The Department of Health – approximately £1 billion a year is allocated to help fund healthcare research projects, mainly through the National Institute for Health Research (NIHR) and the Department of Health's policy research programme.
- Research councils
  - Biotechnology and Biological Sciences Research Council
  - Medical Research Council
- Research charities
  - Welcome Trust
  - The Academy of Medical Sciences
  - Medical Research Foundation
  - The Royal Society
  - British Medical Association
- Think tanks
  - The King's Fund
  - The Nuffield Trust
- Specialty-specific charities
  - Age UK
  - Alzheimer's Research UK
  - Arthritis Research UK
  - British Heart Foundation
  - Cancer Research UK
  - Diabetes UK
  - Stroke Association
- Medical schools
- Hospital research and development departments
- Industry, including pharmaceutical companies
- Private health companies
- Royal colleges and specialty societies

Applications for funding differ depending on the specific funding body you apply to. The majority of funding bodies expect you to fill out an electronic application form, which may be followed by a face-to-face interview in front of a funding panel if shortlisted.

7. While an NIHR pathway for training clinical academics exists, do not be afraid to go outside of medicine to do some additional training in research methods, e.g., BSc, MSc, MD or PhD. It is important to be flexible about the path your career may take.
8. Most importantly, believe in yourself!

ADVICE FOR SOMEONE CONSIDERING A CAREER IN ACADEMIC MEDICINE

1. Find a role model whom you admire, someone who is supportive and understanding and who encourages you to pursue your dreams.
2. Do not rush into the first project that comes your way. It is essential that you use your clinical experience to inform your research interests and look for the right supervisor to support you in achieving your goals. Visit the department before applying for a post.
3. Whether you are making career decisions or carrying out an academic project, do not be afraid to ask for advice.
4. Having established your long-term goals, set short-term objectives to assist you in achieving them. Review your goals regularly. Try and resist taking on too many things at one time.
5. Relish the intellectual challenge and enjoy all steps of the academic process; formulate a clinically relevant question, secure funding and see the project through to the end.
6. Establish strong collaborations with experts in your field of research – collaboration teamwork garners recognition, greater resources and rewards.

Advantages of a career in academic medicine

- Great opportunities to carry out, publish and present cutting-edge research
- Opportunities to travel and lecture abroad
- Can balance research and clinical medicine
- Involves teaching new and old innovations to fellow clinicians and the public
- Associated with great respect in the community

Disadvantages of a career in academic medicine

- Job security is questionable
- Less flexibility in managing your academic or clinical duties than in private practice
- Less clinically skilled than pure clinical doctors, as there is less incentive to see more patients
- Pressure for securing grants can be very high, as you must satisfy your employer
- Meeting deadlines for grant applications or submitting articles can be a huge burden

---

● Chapter Summary

- With many routes to research training at all stages throughout your career, it is never too late to get involved in research.
- Integrated academic training pathways offer formal training in research alongside clinical training.
- There is a wide variety in the types of research and nonresearch activities, as well as the types of research methodologies, that contribute to advancing medical knowledge and practice.
- Identifying and addressing gaps in clinical evidence requires enthusiasm, dedication and collaboration between healthcare professionals.
- A number of factors should be considered when identifying a research project supervisor to guide and support you throughout your research project from inception to publication and presentation.
- Prior to committing to any significant research project, you need to ensure that either the supervisor has adequate funding for you or that they will support you with an application for adequate funding.

FURTHER READING

UK Clinical Research Collaboration, 2005. Medically- and dentally-qualified academic staff: Recommendations for training the researchers and educators of the future (The Walport Report).

Medical Research Council. Funding. Available from: https://www.mrc.ac.uk/funding/ [Accessed 21st September 2018].

National Institute for Health Research. Guide to National Institute for Health Research integrated academic training. Available from: https://www.nihr.ac.uk/funding-and-support/documents/IAT/TCC-NIHR-IAT-GUIDE.pdf [Accessed 21st September 2018].

The Academy of Medical Sciences. Grants and Programmes. Available from: https://acmedsci.ac.uk/grants-and-schemes [Accessed 21st September 2018].

UK Foundation Programme. Academic Foundation Programme. Available from: http://www.foundationprogramme.nhs.uk/content/academic-foundation-programme-0 [Accessed 21st September 2018].

UK Clinical Research Collaboration. Workforce Training. Available from: http://www.ukcrc.org/workforce-training/ [Accessed 21st September 2018].

Wellcome. Funding. Available from https://wellcome.ac.uk/funding [Accessed 21st September 2018].

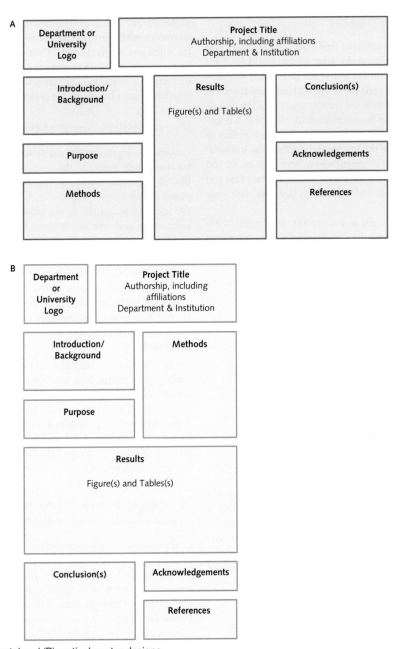

Fig. 4.2 (A) Horizontal and (B) vertical poster designs.

Printing your poster

Once you have completed the first draft of your poster, you must run it by your co-authors for feedback and final approval before you send the poster for printing. If you submit something with their name on, without their approval, and they later object to it, the consequences could be severe, including loss of your license to practice medicine. It is important to get feedback on the design, layout, legibility of the text, resolution of the images and clarity of the information provided. Once all amendments have been made and you are ready to print your poster, it is important that you select the correct size and orientation that you want your poster printed in.

If you study or work at a university or hospital, there should be local printing facility. Printing a large poster can take time, therefore it is important to allow sufficient time, ideally at least 72 hours prior to the deadline. There may be an option to laminate your poster, which involves adding a plastic sheet to give it a shiny effect. There are two main types of lamination:

- Matte finish is useful if your poster has many images that need to look clear. While there is less of a glare, the poster may overall have a dull look.
- Gloss finish is shinier, similar to that of a magazine page, and may therefore be better for posters with fine detail.
- Regardless of the lamination type, it does not protect your poster from scratches, fingerprints or the weather.

It is possible to get your poster printed on materials other than paper, such as cloth; however, it is important that you clarify whether any rules have been set by the conference with regards to acceptable materials for printing. Cloth is sometimes a good option if you have to transport your poster as carry-on luggage on a flight. However, you should note that the weave of the cloth can reduce the apparent resolution of the text and images. This can be particularly harmful if there are photographic images. If you have printed your poster on paper, invest in a sturdy poster tube to prevent it from getting creased or wet during transportation.

COMMON PITFALLS

Double check that your poster is being printed in the same size and orientation as those specifications you designed your poster in.

Poster handout

Most posters are left up for the entire day of the presentation or for the duration of the conference. As you will not be able to stand next to the poster to deliver your presentation at all times, it may be useful to print A4 copies of your poster, ideally in colour. The poster handout can be given to visitors, with spares left in a small bundle near the poster for when you are not present. On the reverse of the poster handout, you may wish to provide your contact details and/or further information such as references to publications which have stemmed from the project.

Presenting your poster

Conference organisers should provide you with a means for fixing your poster to the supplied poster boards. Pins, BluTak or adhesive stickers may be used to secure your poster to the boards. If possible, try to put the poster at eye level. To access the forms, please visit http://www.expertconsult.com. See inside cover for registration details. Conferences usually have a dedicated poster session when you are expected to stand next to your poster. You should be able to deliver two separate summaries of your project:

- A five sentence summary covering the essentials of the project for those visitors with limited time.
- A 2- to 5-minute summary addressing the poster topics in more depth for those who are interested in the project.

Try to smile and be confident and enthusiastic when presenting your poster. It is important to practice your presentation in advance of the conference. A 'best poster' that was presented at an international conference can be viewed online. Many of the principles discussed in this section have been incorporated into the poster. To access this content, please visit http://www.expertconsult.com. See inside cover for registration details.

Oral presentations are commonly used as teaching material, in addition to being an important part of sharing your clinical and research work. In this section we will some discuss generic rules on how to create a dynamic and innovative presentation. Although some of the success in giving an effective presentation lies in the content, the rest lies in the speaker's presentation skills. Similar to poster presentations, it is important to determine if your oral presentation will be 'judged' at the conference. If so, it is important to review the judging criteria, which should be available on the conference website.

Presentation preparation

Microsoft PowerPoint is the most common software used to design slides for an oral presentation. The preparation phase for an oral presentation centres on two key areas:
- Session content
- Slide design

Session content

Content framework

- The first step involves devising a structured framework of the content to be covered in the presentation.
- A decision needs to be made on the session topic, learning goals, learning objectives and the flow of the content material during the course of the presentation.
- For a presentation of a research project, a similar framework should be used as outlined in the 'Content' subsection of the 'Poster preparation' section above. The following sequence of slides should be used:
  - Slide 1: Title, authors and affiliations
  - Slide 2: Conflict of interest statement
  - Slide 3: Introduction/background and purpose
  - Slide 4: Methods
  - Slide 5: Results
  - Slide 6: Conclusions
  - Slide 7: Acknowledgements or funding
  - Slide 8: References
  - Slide 9: Any questions?

The methods and results sections are usually longer than the others, and may require more than one slide each.

- For nonresearch presentations, once the headings of your content framework have been transferred into your PowerPoint presentation, do not feel you are tied down to your initial sequence.

HINTS AND TIPS

When preparing a PowerPoint presentation, the framework or storyboard should be decided first before thinking about the text, colour, layout, audio or video.

Creativity

- In this part of the preparation process, you need to link your own creativity with the learning objectives for the presentation.
- The following should be clarified:
  - Illustrations – e.g., flowcharts, graphs and pictures.
  - An illustration is worth a thousand words, and is usually more interesting than text. There are reports suggesting that people generally remember 20% of what they hear, 30% of what they see and 50% of what they see and hear. If you borrowed an illustration from another source, avoid any copyright infringement by acknowledging your source. If a patient can be identified from a photograph taken at a clinical setting, a signed form by the patient granting permission for use is required.
  - Animations – Movement of text or images on screen can attract attention, but complex animations should be avoided.
  - Video – Some people try to avoid videos due to concerns regarding the video failing to run or being too slow to play. Others are confused about whether to embed a video file (so that it becomes a permanent part of the presentation) or link a video (from an internet site or from a separate computer file) to the PowerPoint presentation. Table 4.1 summarizes the advantages and disadvantages of both approaches to incorporating a video into a PowerPoint presentation.
  - Sounds – If you wish to include sound clips or audio files, it is important to make sure that the computer output will be connected to an amplifier on the day of your presentation.

Slide design

- If you are feeling adventurous, you can create your own slide design from scratch.
- There are predesigned master slide templates that allow you to fill in titles and add text and graphics to the slide.

Table 4.1 Video files: to link or not to link, to embed or not to embed?

	Advantages	Disadvantages
Linking a video file	– Presentation file size kept to a minimum. – Video from anywhere on the internet can be used, so that it is current.	– If using your own videos, you must always make sure the video file is copied along with the presentation file if the slides are to be viewed on another computer. – For online videos, an internet connection is required during the presentation, which is not offered at all venues (check in advance!)
Embedding a video file	– The embedded video becomes a permanent part of the presentation, just like the illustrations and animations. – One single file is created which can be shared amongst colleagues or easily viewed on another computer.	– The final file size can become relatively large. – The presentation might grind to a halt if the computer running the file is overwhelmed by the file size. This is more of an issue if your computer is not a fairly recent model.

- Words should be in contrast to the background, either dark-coloured words on a light-coloured background or vice versa.
- It is important to try to avoid clashing colour schemes.
- Keep the colour schemes constant throughout the presentation.
- Try to avoid red text, as it has been reported that colour blindness affects approximately 10% of men of European origin, with red-green colour blindness being the most common form.
- Ideally, only five bullet points should be used on a single slide.
- Font size decisions will depend on the size of the presentation room; however, a minimum font size of 24 is recommended.
- Use capital letters for abbreviations; otherwise, they should be used sparingly.
- Use common, easy-to-read fonts such as Arial, Calibri or Helvetica.
- A prize-winning PowerPoint presentation that was presented at an international conference can be viewed online. Many of the principles discussed in this section have been incorporated into the slides. To access this content, please visit http://www.expertconsult.com. See inside cover for registration details. The following section will focus on how to deliver your presentation, which also plays a role in how oral presentations are judged.

COMMON PITFALLS

It is important to perform a spell check once you have completed your slides. Most software packages such as PowerPoint distinguish not only languages, but variants, so it is worth specifying to the spellcheck software that the language is, for example, UK English or US English.

HINTS AND TIPS

Once you have created your slides, rehearse your presentation in front of at least one person, requesting feedback and amending the presentation accordingly. If possible, practise the presentation in the venue itself so that things are familiar on the day of the actual presentation.

Presenting your slides

Setting the stage

Most people will not be giving their presentation from the same computer used to design their slides. When transferring your PowerPoint presentation, it is important to save it using at least two different approaches, including saving it on a USB stick, emailing it to yourself or uploading it on to an online file sharing and storage platform such as Dropbox. As highlighted above, if you have a video file that is linked to your presentation, this also needs to be transferred. You must prepare for the worst eventuality, and having multiple backups of your presentation is advisable.

If you are going to use your own laptop to run your presentation, it is important to ensure prior to the presentation day that the venue has the appropriate cables and connections to attach your computer to the projector. Once your equipment is ready and your presentation is uploaded, run through the slides, if possible. Use the 'speaker ready room', if one is available. Before you start the presentation, you can set it to 'presenter view', which has the following features:

- Preview text: this shows what the next click will add to the screen; for example, a new bullet point, a new illustration illustration or the next slide.
- Speaker's notes: this is shown in large, clear font, and can be used as a prompt or script for the presentation. The notes can be written for each slide when you design your slides.

Delivering the presentation

Every presentation should be treated as a performance. This involves knowing the lines of your presentation and the related subject area. It is not recommended to present a completely memorized presentation, as this can end up sounding unnatural or you may end up unsettled by any interruptions. During your practice sessions, you should focus on memorizing the key points you wish to make (noting them down in the 'speaker notes' section, if this may help) and subsequently improvise different various ways of communicating the message. While fear of public speaking is common, a number of simple strategies can be employed to help manage these fears:

- Calm your nerves by breathing slowly and deeply for a few moments before the start of your presentation.
- Affirm to yourself that you are relaxed and confident.
- Try to visualize yourself give a relaxed presentation.
- Whether the last two points are effective techniques is debatable, but you won't know unless you try!

When your name is called to give your presentation, enthusiastically walk up to the podium. You should stand tall, keep your chest lifted and smile! There is research to show that smiling reduces stress. You would rather listen to someone who is smiling than someone who comes across as overly stern and boring! A microphone should be used if one is available; otherwise, try to project your voice from your diaphragm rather than from your throat. It is important to talk to the audience to help you connect with them, rather than talking to the screen by reading from your slides. You should pace yourself to ensure that you stick to the allocated time frame given for your talk. At the end of the presentation, thank the audience for listening and open the floor to any questions they may have about the talk.

HINTS AND TIPS

When preparing your slides and rehearsing your performance, make a note of the slide you should be presenting midway through your talk. This slide should act as a benchmark for letting you know whether there is a need to slow down or speed up the remainder of the presentation.

ANSWERING AUDIENCE QUESTIONS

By and large, audiences are well-behaved and supportive. They do not usually see the value in questioning-as-a-blood-sport. The question and answer section of the presentation is a chance for dialogue. It is important to appreciate that it is not a test or a viva! No one knows your project better than you, therefore be confident, and you will be able to answer your questions with ease! Be reassured that the majority of people from the audience who ask questions are doing so out of genuine interest. They either want more information about your project or they want to flag some relevant information which you may not be aware of. If you know the answer to a question asked, say it as succinctly as you can, taking a moment or two to compose your answer before you start speaking. If someone offers you new information, then thank them, helpful or not! There are a few scenarios which may warrant a specific approach:

- The question with no clear answer
- The paternalistic questioner
- The questioner who keeps on questioning
- The hostile questioner

The question with no clear answer

If you are asked a question that you do not know the answer to, it is important to acknowledge that you are not sure of the answer and will need to do some additional reading and/or perform a new study to get an answer, rather than trying to cobble something together. You do not need to have an immediate answer to every question. Sometimes asking the questioner to elaborate further on their question may not only lead to you getting more information and bide more time for you to work out the answer, but may even lead to the questioner answering their own question!

The paternalistic questioner

As a student or junior doctor, you may find that the experienced researcher may decide to 'school' you by giving you some supervision or advice, rather than specifically asking you any questions. Whilst this can be irritating, the best response is to smile and thank them for their thoughts, rather than to confront their paternalistic behaviour. Others in the audience are likely to appreciate what is happening and feel your frustration.

The questioner that keeps on questioning

Prolonged two-person interaction may lead to others in the audience getting bored, therefore this should be avoided. If you find yourself in this situation, you should suggest that you stop the dialogue and continue your conversation after the session, allowing other people from the audience a chance to ask questions.

The hostile questioner

Occasionally, there may be someone in the audience who is rude or aggressive. Despite the nonspecific criticism, you need to stay polite, smile and acknowledge their contribution. Asking for more information may generate useful discussion. Alternatively, another audience member, such as your supervisor, may come to your 'rescue'. Another approach is to invite other members of the audience for their input by asking them what they feel about the comments made.

HINTS AND TIPS

It is important to rehearse what you are going to say during your presentation. If you are worried about the question and answer session, you could arrange with one of your friends to ask a question that you know that you can answer well. Arranging for them to ask you the first question may help settle your nerves. Another option is to ask your supervisor to step in and mind your back if you find yourself struggling during the question and answer session.

HINTS AND TIPS

The session chair has a responsibility to ask a question if nobody in the audience asks one. This can be onerous for them, and they may appreciate it if you introduce yourself beforehand and say that you are 'hoping that somebody will ask X, because this will lead to an interesting discussion'. That allows them to relax and enjoy your presentation rather than feeling continuous pressure to think of a question to ask.

Chapter Summary

- Presentations at local meetings or at national or international conferences aid in the dissemination of your findings.
- Choosing the right meeting or conference for abstract submission remains a crucial step in the submission process.
- Abstract submissions are usually made online, with very specific instructions and strict rules about word limit, font and space size.
- If your abstract is accepted for a poster presentation, the poster specification, layout and content should all be considered during the preparation process.
- When presenting a poster, you need to be able to deliver two separate summaries of your project:
  - A five sentence summary covering the essentials of the project for those visitors with limited time.
  - A 2- to-5-minute summary addressing the poster topics in more depth for those who are interested in the project.
- If your abstract is accepted for an oral presentation, the slide content framework, slide design and various creative elements should all be considered during the preparation process.
- All oral presentations should be treated as a performance. During your practice sessions, you should focus on memorizing the key points you wish to make, and subsequently improvise different various ways of communicating the message.
- The question and answer section of a presentation is a chance for dialogue. It is important to appreciate that it is not a test or a viva!

FURTHER READING

Bourne, P.E., 2007. Ten simple rules for making good oral presentations. PLoS Comput. Biol. 3 (4), e77.

Larkin M. How to give a dynamic scientific presentation. Available from: https://www.elsevier.com/connect/how-to-give-a-dynamic-scientific-presentation [Accessed 21st September 2018].

Miller, J.E., 2007. Preparing and presenting effective research posters. Health Serv. Res. 42, 311–328.

you make your final choice, you could consider the following questions:

- In a rush to publish? Some journals offer rapid publication.
- Highest impact factor? You could simply submit the manuscript to the journal which has the highest impact factor. Be realistic, however!
- Highest publication acceptance rate? Some journals with good impact factors have higher acceptance rates than others. Most journal websites state their manuscript submission acceptance rates.
- Reach as many readers as possible? Some journals provide an open access option, which allows anyone to read your article, free of charge, online. This may improve the chances of the article being read and subsequently cited, if accepted. This may come at a fee, however!

HINTS AND TIPS

While you may believe that your research project is of utmost importance to the medical community, you must objectively consider the significance of your results in your field of research. You need to ask yourself: 'What are the implications of my results?'. This will help you evaluate the overall impact of your research and what journal it may be best suited for.

HINTS AND TIPS

During the process of deciding which journal to submit your manuscript to, consider emailing the editor of your preferred journal choice with the key messages of your research to determine whether your paper is appropriate for submission to their journal.

Instructions for authors

Each journal has a very different approach to how they publish their research articles, therefore it is advisable that you read the journal-specific 'instructions for authors'. To maximize the chances of your paper being accepted, it is important that you review and follow the instructions for authors section very carefully. The publisher of the journal reserves the right to return manuscripts that have not been prepared in accordance with the instructions provided. The instructions include information on a range of factors, including:

- General considerations, e.g., abbreviations, SI units (International System of Units), etc.

- Research manuscript sections
- Referencing style
- Formatting guidelines
- Preparing figures and tables
- Guidelines for web extra material
- Data deposit
- Publication ethics
- Statements and permissions

Following these guidelines will ensure the editors and reviewers have a much easier job considering your paper, making the process as efficient as possible.

Cover letter

The cover letter gives you an opportunity to 'sell' your manuscript to the editor of the journal. The letter allows you to introduce your work and explain why the manuscript will be of interest to the journal's readers. Initially, you should check to see whether the journal's instructions for authors section lists any cover letter requirements, e.g., statements, disclosures, potential manuscript reviewers. The following structure covers the key points that should be included in your cover letter:

- As with any type of letter, put your address in the top right hand corner of the page, with today's date underneath.
- Address the editor-in-chief who will be assessing your manuscript by their name, e.g., Dear Professor Francis.
- First paragraph: Introduce the title of the manuscript and the type of article you are submitting (e.g., case report, review, research). The background to the study should be explained, as well as the question you sought to answer (and why).
- Second paragraph: Provide a brief explanation of what was done during your study and the main study findings. Explain why the results are significant in the relevant field of medicine or surgery.
- Third paragraph: Explain why the target audience of the journal would be interested in your paper. The aims and scope of the journal may provide useful cues to help you with this statement.
- Conclude your letter with any journal specific requirements, e.g., statements, disclosures, potential manuscript reviewers. You will need to make a note of any potential 'overlapping' content submitted or accepted to another journal or conference.
- Finally, you should state: 'All authors have read and approved the submitted manuscript, and the manuscript has not been submitted elsewhere nor published elsewhere in whole or in part, except as an abstract (if relevant).'
- Finish your letter formally: 'Thank you for your consideration of this manuscript', followed by 'Yours sincerely', and then print and sign your name at the bottom.

A cover letter which was previously used for an accepted manuscript can be viewed online. To access this content, please visit http://www.expertconsult.com. See inside cover for registration details.

Presubmission checklist

In order to reduce the chance of your manuscript being returned to you before reaching the editor, you should check the following:

- Author information: All coauthor details should be provided.
- Manuscript length and formatting: The manuscript should not exceed the requirements for word count, number of tables and/or figures and number of references. Any additional information for your article type should be provided, such as 'key messages'.
- Tables/figures: All tables and/or figures should have appropriate legends and be cited in the text. When using a graph to plot your data, remember to ensure that both the x- and y-axis are labelled, where relevant. The figures should also be uploaded in the recommended file format and be of sufficient quality for potential publication.
- References: All the references should be cited in the text and formatted using the recommended referencing system (e.g., Vancouver style, Harvard style).
- Supplementary files: Any supplementary files should be supplied in the accepted file format and cited in the main text.
- Statements: Necessary statements about contributorship, competing interests, funding, data sharing, patient consent and ethical approval should be provided.
- Research reporting checklists: You may be required to provide an appropriate statement for your study type, e.g., CONSORT (Consolidated Standards of Reporting Trials) guidelines for randomised controlled trials (Chapter 11), PRISMA (Preferred Reporting Items for Systematic Reviews and Meta-Analyses) guidelines for systematic reviews and meta-analyses (Chapter 9).
- Reviewers: You should provide the names of preferred and nonpreferred reviewers, if this is required as part of the submission process.

DEALING WITH A REJECTED MANUSCRIPT

Submitting your article to a journal is only the first step in the process to getting it published. Most journals will require at the very least some amendments based on the feedback received from the journal editor and reviewers. It is very rare that a journal will accept an article without amendment from the author(s).

Responding to reviewer and editor comments

There are different types of verdicts that a journal will use. They may differ slightly in terminology; however, the following list is fairly typical:

- Reject outright without review
- Reject outright following review
- Reconsider after major revision (no indication of likelihood of acceptance)
- Reconsider after minor revision (likely to accept eventually)
- Accept

We will focus on the two outcomes (3 and 4) in which there are still opportunities for the manuscript to be accepted. The journal will send you a full list of comments from each reviewer along with the editor's verdict. The next step is to address the comments from the editor and each of the reviewers to ensure your paper is reconsidered and has the best opportunity of being accepted.

Understanding the comments

The comments should be read carefully to ensure that you understand the points that have been raised. While you may disagree with some of the comments, you should not take them personally. Remember, they are meant to help you improve your paper. If you are unclear about any of the comments, you should discuss them with your coauthors before writing to the journal editor for further explanation. You may be faced with a situation where two different reviewers have provided comments that contradict each other. In this situation, you need to use your judgement and consult your coauthors, explaining clearly in your response as to why you opted one way than the other.

Responding to every comment

You need to think about every comment and how you wish to respond, following consultation with all coauthors. A 'response to reviewer' document should be prepared with clear and concise responses showing your changes or reasons why certain comments have been dealt with in a particular way. Rather than referring to comments ('Refer to "Comment 1, Reviewer 1"'), you should copy and paste each comment into a new document. Each individual reviewer comment should be followed by an author comment clearly explaining any suggestions you disagree with and why. You must be diplomatic in your responses and provide evidence to back up your thought process. You should make a clear reference as to where changes have been made in the revised manuscript, as well as copying them in to your response to reviewer document. Remaining positive, polite and concise are key factors to remember. For example, here is how we responded to a couple of the reviewer comments received for the following published paper:

- Kaura A, Sunderland N, Kamdar R, Petzer E, Murgatroyd F, Dhillon P, Scott P. Identifying patients with less potential to benefit from implantable cardioverter-defibrillator therapy: comparison of the performance of four risk scoring systems. *J Interv Card Electrophysiol* 2017; 49(2):181–189.

Reviewer 1, Comment 1
If the data are available, it would be useful to analyse cause of death in this study, to see if cause of death differs between patients with low versus high risk scores using the various scoring systems.

Authors' Response
We agree with the reviewer that it would be interesting to assess the association between the scoring systems and mode/cause of death. Unfortunately, due to the retrospective observational nature of this analysis, this data is not available.

Reviewer 1, Comment 2
On page 10, the authors describe the rate of appropriate and inappropriate shocks in patients who died within 1 year of ICD implantation. It would be useful to analyse the appropriate and inappropriate shock rate in all patients in this study, and to determine whether the scoring systems used to predict mortality are also predictive of appropriate and inappropriate shocks. This could help to better determine the likelihood of ICD benefit in these patients.

Authors' Response
As suggested by the reviewer we have analysed the relationship between the scoring systems and the occurrence of appropriate/inappropriate ICD therapy. We have added an extra table (Table 7) and some extra text in the results section.

Changes Made
Page 7
2.3. Statistical Analysis
Cox proportional hazards regression modelling was used to evaluate the relationship between each scoring system and the occurrence of appropriate and inappropriate ICD therapy during follow-up.

Page 10
Relationship of Scoring Systems to Device Therapy
During follow-up, 106 (26.1%) patients experienced appropriate device therapy (36 ATP, 30 shock and 40 ATP followed by shock) and 38 (9.4%) patients inappropriate therapy (18

ATP, 12 shock and 8 ATP followed by shock). In univariate cox regression analyses, only the Kramer scoring system was associated with the occurrence of appropriate device therapy (hazard ratio 3.15, p=0.003) (Table 7). None of the scoring systems were associated with the occurrence of inappropriate therapy.

Meeting the deadline

The majority of journals have specific deadlines for receiving revised manuscripts. You should plan your response to ensure that you have given yourself enough time to revise your manuscript, write the response to reviewers and have them both reviewed by all coauthors prior to submission. It is important to not underestimate the time required to make changes, especially if you need to revisit or reanalyse data or add additional content.

Submitting to an alternative journal

There are several reasons why a submission may be rejected, from insufficient scientific rigor to poor language quality. It is possible that your manuscript was turned down, not due to issues with the research methodology or scientific rigor per se, but due to the topic area being out of the scope with the aims of the journal to which it was submitted. In this situation, you need to search for a journal that has an appropriate aim and scope to warrant publication of your findings.

Your paper may have been rejected outright or rejected after failing to satisfy the reviewer comments followed a revised manuscript submission. In this situation, you should not just send the original version of the manuscript to another journal, as it is possible that the second journal will give a similar verdict (after possibly even using the same reviewers, if they are experts in the particular field of your project area!). You should use all the feedback you have received as an opportunity to revise your paper before you decide on what steps to take next. While your natural instinct is to submit a revised and improved manuscript to a journal with a lower impact factor, according to research from Elsevier, 22% of rejected manuscripts end up being published in a journal with an impact factor equal to or higher than that of the journal to which it was originally submitted. This is somewhat unsurprising, as authors usually use rejection as an opportunity to improve the manuscript before submitting the upgraded paper to a new journal. Just remember not to take rejection personally, and keep trying!

Chapter Summary

- There are a number of elements involved in a written report of a research study:
  - Title: presents a highly condensed version of the abstract
  - Abstract: helps readers discern whether they are interested (or not) in reading the research report
  - Introduction: discusses the rationale behind the study
  - Methods: documents all the methods used in your study so that a reader would know exactly how to repeat the study
  - Results: present and illustrate your findings
  - Discussion: provides an interpretation of your results, using evidence from the literature to make your conclusions
  - References: acknowledges all sources of information referred to in the research paper
- A number of factors should be considered when choosing which journal to submit your manuscript to, including clarifying its reputation and target audience.
- Each journal has a very different approach to how they publish their research articles, therefore it is advisable that you read the journal-specific instructions for authors.
- The cover letter gives you an opportunity to 'sell' your manuscript to the editor of the journal. A clear structure should be used when constructing your letter.
- Following submission of your manuscript to a journal, you will subsequently receive a full list of comments from each reviewer along with the editor's verdict. If your paper requires minor or major revisions, the next step is to handle the comments from the editor and each of the reviewers to ensure your paper is reconsidered and has the best opportunity of being accepted.

FURTHER READING

Giuseppe, L., 2017. How do I write a scientific article? – A personal perspective. Ann. Transl. Med. 5 (20), 416.

Hall, G. (Ed.), 2012. How to Write a Paper, fifth ed. BMJ Publishing Group, London.

Quinn, C.T., Rush, A.J., 2009. Writing and publishing your research findings. J. Investig. Med. 57 (5), 634–639.

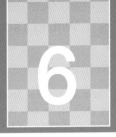

Writing a successful curriculum vitae

6

IS A CURRICULUM VITAE NECESSARY?

A curriculum vitae (CV) may be required at any part of your medical career, from your medical school elective through to a registrar or consultant post, or when applying for a postgraduate degree such as a PhD or an MD. Your CV is a vital resource that can be referred to when completing an application form, and can be used for networking purposes. It should be part of your professional portfolio, a physical folder of evidence of the achievements included in your CV.

WHAT IS A CURRICULUM VITAE?

A CV is a record of your personal, educational and work achievements. It should be viewed as a marketing tool to help convince the reader that you have the necessary skills and experience. There is no such thing as a 'general' CV; most effective CVs are those that are tailored to the specific requirements of a job or course. Before you start writing your CV, it is important that you read the person specification (for a job) or the entry requirements (for a degree). The criteria listed will be used to make an assessment of who should be shortlisted for an interview. The person specification or entry requirements may give you a clue as to how your CV should be tailored.

A good first impression of your CV is crucial, therefore it is important to make it as relevant and as clear as possible. You may choose to emphasize certain aspects of your skills and experiences over others, in accordance with the person specification or entry requirements. Other sources of information to help you identify the desirable skills and experience expected may include speaking to previous successful applicants or reading the online information provided by the institution beyond the person specification or entry requirements. In order to tailor your CV, you need to subsequently think about specific examples that best demonstrate your skills and experience in accordance with what is required for the post or degree. These examples should not only cover prior employment, clinical skills and academic skills, but also leisure activities and interests such as sporting achievements.

HINTS AND TIPS

You should revise your CV for each job or degree application, rather than submitting a generic version on every occasion.

WRITING AN EFFECTIVE CURRICULUM VITAE

There are no definitive rules on how to write your CV, and no official templates to follow. The General Medical Council (GMC) provide brief guidance on what to include in a CV. We will elaborate on this information and cover some key conventions that should be followed when writing an effective medical CV. A model CV template can be viewed online. To access this content, please visit http://www.expertconsult.com. See inside cover for registration details.

Curriculum vitae length

Due to the nature of the profession, medical CVs can be notoriously long. The length of your CV is likely to be reflective of the number of years of service:

- Medical student/junior doctor: 2–3 pages
- Senior doctor/registrar: 4–5 pages
- Consultant: 7–8 pages
- Academic: 30–50 pages

If you have many pages of publications or presentations, it is better to add them as an appendix at the end of the CV.

HINTS AND TIPS

Readers appreciate a short CV that begins with what is most impressive to them. If you wish to start with certain sections for impact, feel free to do so.

Front sheet

There are different opinions on whether a cover page should be included or not. We recommend not having a front sheet, because when the CV is sitting on the table in front of the interviewer, there is nothing advantageous being conveyed to them by your name and the title 'CV' - unless your name is Einstein! If you still wish to include one, the front sheet could cover the following details:

- Title and full name, e.g., Dr John Doe
- Credentials, e.g., MB ChB, BSc
- The name of the post or degree you are applying for, if necessary
- Job reference number, if necessary

Structure

We recommend the following ordered structure for a medical CV:

1. Personal details and contact information
2. Professional registration
3. Memberships
4. Career aim*
5. Qualifications
6. Prizes and awards
7. Employment history 1 – posts held
8. Employment history 2 – gaps in employment
9. Research experience
10. Publications
11. Presentations
12. Conferences
13. Courses/continuing professional development (CPD)
14. Audit and quality improvement
15. Teaching and training experience
16. Management and leadership experience
17. Skills and experience
18. Extra activities/personal interests
19. References*

All of the sections above have been listed by the GMC. The asterisk (*) denotes additional sections we recommend.

Personal details and contact information

The following sections should be included:

- Name: This should match the name indicated on your proof of identity and should be in large font. The other items could all be placed on one or two lines, in a small font. They do not contribute to you getting the job.
- Address
- Nationality (including visa status, if relevant)
- Telephone number: In the modern era, readers expect to see the mobile number. Only give additional numbers if your home or office number has an answer machine and your mobile does not.
- E-mail address: Avoid casual or embarrassing addresses, e.g., partydoc@xxx.com. It may also be worth avoiding addresses tied to a particular institution, because you may lose access in the future.
- The previous convention was to include gender, date of birth or age and marital status. In the modern era, these open the way to unfair discrimination, and therefore are usually not put on a CV.

The contact information on your CV should match the details that you have provided to the GMC (which can be updated on the GMC website).

Professional registration

The following sections should be included:

- GMC reference number
- Date of entry to the specialist register, if relevant
- National Training Number, if relevant

Memberships

List your membership of professional bodies, including year of membership commencement. The memberships should be listed in chronological order from most recent, working backwards.

Career aim

This section can also be entitled 'Career goal' or 'Career objective'. It is becoming increasingly common to see CVs that start with a short personal statement. This should be no longer than 5–6 lines. The statement should, in a nutshell, outline the key skills and experiences you have that make you the best candidate for the post or degree you have applied for. You should also include a sentence or two on how the post or degree fits into your short-term and long-term goals.

Qualifications

List all of your qualifications in reverse chronological order, along with the relevant dates and place of study. If your A-level or GCSE results are unusually good, do not feel embarrassed to list them one by one with their grades, since this shows a long track record of systematically delivering across a broad range of areas. You should also list any qualifications you are currently studying for, e.g., membership exams, medical education degree, etc. These can be displayed in a table, with date of completion or commencement (for ongoing degrees) in the left-hand column, qualification in the second column and place of study in the third column.

Prizes and awards

List any prizes or awards (with dates) in reverse chronological order, along with a description and who granted it. You should also include the number of people you competed against for each award, if known. Use a tabular format, with date in the first column and title of prize, awarding body and description (including number of people eligible for the award) all listed on separate lines in the second column.

Employment history 1 – posts held

List your employment history in reverse chronological order, with the following information:

- Post title
- Dates (DD/MM/YYYY – DD/MM/YYYY)
- If the post was part-time, what percentage of whole time equivalent
- Institution name and location (e.g., Hammersmith Hospital, London, UK)
- Name of your clinical supervisor
- A brief job description that covers the duties (experience, clinical skills and procedures) required for the post

For the brief job description, you should consider the following points:

- You should focus on highlighting the clinical skills and experiences that are most relevant to the post or degree that you are currently applying for.
- The clinical skills and experiences may include inpatient work, outpatient work, dealing with particular types of emergencies and procedural/surgical experience.
- If you have held a number of posts, to avoid repetition, you could list your skills and experiences across several similar level posts, e.g., foundation year 1, senior house offer and registrar positions.
- To allow the interviewers to be able to pick out the essential information more efficiently, use bullet points, not complete sentences.

If you are a specialist trainee or consultant, rather than writing a brief job description for each of the posts unrelated to your practicing specialty, you should complete the section below (Section 17: Skills and experience).

COMMON PITFALLS

You should try to avoid personal, reflective statements such as 'I had a really good time on this post as I had the opportunity to…'. Only facts should be included in your CV; there will be an opportunity to provide reflective statements during the face-to-face interview if you are shortlisted.

Employment history 2 – gaps in employment

Gaps in employment are any time periods greater than 28 days during which you were not employed. These should be accounted for with a brief explanation. This section is usually only relevant when applying for training posts such as core training, registrar or consultant posts. If applicable, you should list these in a reverse chronological order.

Research experience

In reverse chronological order, you should quote the title of your research project, along with the dates of when it was undertaken and the name of your supervisor. You should also provide a brief description of your specific role in the project, in bullet point format. This information should be displayed in a table with the date in the first column and the title of your project, a brief description of the project and the name of your supervisor on separate lines in the second column. As you gain more research experience, you may move this section in to an appendix at the end of the CV.

Publications

Many people present their publications in the conventional manner, i.e., Vancouver style (please refer to Chapter 5), where author names are first, followed by the tittle of the publication and then the journal. The issue with this approach is that the titles of the different projects will be all over the place on the page, which will make it more difficult for an interviewer to locate and therefore appreciate the various topics that you have worked on. A more common approach is to present your publications in a tabular format, with the year of publication in the left-hand column, followed by a column with the title, the authors and the journal, each on separate lines. The publications should be listed in reverse chronological order. To improve readability, you can categorize your publications into the following categories:

- Peer-reviewed journals
- Books
- Book chapters
- Abstracts

If you have a relatively long list of publications, consider moving the publications to an appendix at the end of the CV.

Presentations

Similar to the approach with listing your publications, the presentations should be presented in a tabular format to improve readability. The date of presentation should be in the left-hand column, followed by a column with the title, the authors who contributed towards the presentation and the conference or meeting you presented at, each on separate lines. If you have given many presentations, you should categorize them into the following categories:

- International
- National
- Regional
- Departmental

Conferences

All conferences you have attended during the previous five years should be listed in reverse chronological order. For readability, present this in a tabular format with the date of attendance in the left-hand column, the title of the conference and the name of the organizing institution/body in the second column, each listed on separate lines. If you have attended many conferences, you should categorize them into the following categories to improve readability and to show their relative importance:

- International
- National
- Regional
- Departmental

Courses/continuing professional development

The GMC suggests having separate sections for courses and CPD-accredited activities. The main issue with this approach is that many of the courses you attend will be CPD-accredited. We therefore suggest combining the two sections, unless you have a list of CPD activities which were not courses. All courses you have attended from the previous five years should be listed in reverse chronological order. For readability, present this in a tabular format with the date of attendance in the left-hand column, and the title of the course, the name of the organizing institution and the number of CPD points awarded (if relevant) in the second column, all listed on separate lines. If you have attended a diverse range of courses, you may want to categorize them into the following categories, if appropriate:

- Clinical
- Research
- Management
- Teaching

We suggest leaving out all courses which relate to exam preparation, as they do not add any value.

Audit and quality improvement

All audits and quality improvement projects should be listed in reverse chronological order. Present this in a tabular format with the date of the audit or quality improvement project in the left-hand column, and the following listed in the second column:

- Title of project
- Location: the institution at which the project was undertaken
- Aim: reason behind the audit
- Role: your role in the audit
- Results: any conclusions drawn
- Changes: any changes in practice

If you have participated in multiple audits and quality improvement projects, you could list them in separate sections titled 'Audits' and 'Quality improvement projects'.

Teaching and training experience

All teaching or training that you have delivered should be listed in reverse chronological order. Similar to the other sections, the information should be covered in a tabular format with the date of the teaching session delivered in the left-hand column. The following should be listed in the second column:

- Title of teaching session
- Location: the institution at which the teaching was delivered
- Audience: level of experience of audience (e.g., undergraduate or postgraduate) and number of attendees
- Teaching methods: this may include lectures, small-group teaching sessions, simulation training, etc. (please refer to Chapter 28 for a discussion of the different types of teaching methods)

Management and leadership experience

In light of the Medical Leadership Competency Framework, doctors must show management and leadership experience at all stages of their training. Examples of managing people and resources include:

- Designing rotas
- Writing and implementing local protocols or guidelines
- Representing colleagues on a committee, e.g., trainee clinical representative or mess president

Again, the information should be presented in a tabular format, with the dates covering your role in the first column and the following information listed in the second column:

- Title of management or leadership experience
- Location: the institution at which the experience was undertaken
- One to two sentences on your specific role

Skills and experience

Any future employer will be interested to know what skills you have to offer. Any particular person specification requirements should be addressed. An account of your skills and experience can be subdivided, depending on your speciality of practice:

Anaesthetics
- General anaesthetics
- Intensive care
- Outpatient, including types of clinics (e.g., preoperative, pain clinic)
- Procedures, e.g., central venous access, chest drain, intubation

Cardiology
- Inpatient
- Outpatient, including types of clinics (general, interventional, electrophysiology, rapid access chest pain)
- Imaging, e.g., echocardiography, cardiac computed tomography
- Procedures, e.g., angiograms, pacemakers, temporary pacing wires

General medicine
- Inpatient
- Outpatient, including types of clinics
- Procedures, e.g., central venous access, pleural aspiration, chest drain

Obstetrics and gynaecology
- Obstetrics
- Gynaecology
- Outpatient, including types of clinics
- Theatre experience

Paediatrics
- General paediatrics
- Neonatal
- Paediatric intensive care unit
- Outpatient, including types of clinics

Psychiatry
- General adult psychiatry
- Substance misuse
- Outreach
- Psychotherapy
- Outpatient, including types of clinics

Surgery
- General surgery (if you have performed many different types of operations, it may be wiser to include a log book in the appendix)
- Specialist surgery

Table 6.1 Action verbs

Type of action	Action verbs
Clinical skills and experience	- Gained experience of the management of patients with… - Gained exposure to… - Performed - Trained
Set up	- Designed - Developed - Devised - Established - Founded - Led
Made better	- Increased - Improved - Innovated - Recommended - Reduced - Revised - Saved - Transformed
Found out	- Assessed - Analysed - Designed - Identified - Researched - Tested
Communicated/ showed how	- Advised - Directed - Guided - Presented - Performed - Taught - Trained

- Outpatient, including types of clinics
- Under each of these headings you need to describe the extent of your experience, using bullet points.
- Action verbs (Table 6.1) and active wording should be used to describe your skills and experience:
  - Responsible for…
  - Confident in…
  - Proficient in…
- Avoid personal reflections such as 'I really enjoyed this clinical placement because…'.

Extra activities/personal interests

Mention any involvement in voluntary work and list your main hobbies. You should try to include both lone and group activities, using this as an opportunity to highlight any transferable skills such as teamwork, leadership and management.

References

You need to list the number of referees that were requested (usually two or three). It is important to ask for permission from potential referees before you list them on your CV. It is customary to use referees from your two or three most recent training posts if you are a junior doctor. Many job applications request that you list at least one clinical and one academic consultant. In addition to providing their name, you need to provide complete contact information, including place of work, email address and contact numbers.

STYLE AND FORMATTING

Legible, conventional fonts (Arial or Times New Roman) in a normal size (font size 11 or 12) with normal sized margins (1 inch on each side) should be used. Bold, italics and underlining can be used for emphasis; however, they should be used sparingly. Bullet points can be used to highlight key points in a short and precise manner. Bullet points or sentences should start with a verb to get straight to the point, e.g., led, presented, trained, etc. Table 6.1 lists different types of action verbs you could use, depending on the activity concerned. There should be plenty of white space to make the CV easier to follow, rather than trying to cram everything on to one page. Tables used to format information neatly in to columns should not have a border. Each page of your CV should be numbered and have your surname and initials (at the top of each page).

COMMON MISTAKES

The most common errors made with your CV are as follows:

- out of date
- spelling and grammatical errors
- insufficient information is provided
- the structure is not suitable
- has information which does not match the details submitted online, e.g., post dates, job titles, hospital names or supervising consultants.

HINTS AND TIPS

After you have written your CV for the first time, maintaining it should be relatively straightforward. Every new academic and clinical achievement should be added to the relevant section as it happens.

● Chapter Summary

- Your CV is a vital resource that can be referred to when completing an application form, and can be used for networking purposes.
- There is no such thing as a 'general' CV; the most effective CVs are those that are tailored to the specific requirements of a job or course.
- Your CV should follow an ordered, logical structure and have a clear and consistent layout throughout.

FURTHER READING

British Medical Association. Tips for your medical CV. Available from: https://www.bma.org.uk/advice/career/applying-for-a-job/medical-cv [Accessed 21st September 2018].

General Medical Council. Structuring your CV for a specialist or GP registration application. Available from: https://www.gmc-uk.org/registration-and-licensing/join-the-register/registration-applications/structuring-your-cv-for-a-specialist-or-gp-registration-application [Accessed 21st September 2018].

RESEARCH METHODOLOGY

Chapter 7

Handling data 45

Chapter 8

Investigating hypotheses. 61

Chapter 9

Systematic review and meta-analysis 77

Chapter 10

Research design 89

Chapter 11

Randomized controlled trials. 97

Chapter 12

Cohort studies 115

Chapter 13

Case–control studies. 125

Chapter 14

Measures of disease occurrence and
cross-sectional studies. 137

Chapter 15

Ecological studies 149

Chapter 16

Case report and case series 157

Chapter 17

Qualitative research 161

Chapter 18

Confounding 167

Chapter 19

Screening, diagnosis and prognosis 173

Chapter 20

Statistical techniques 191

Chapter 21

Economic evaluation 199

Chapter 22

Critical appraisal checklists 215

Chapter 23

Crash course in statistical formulae 221

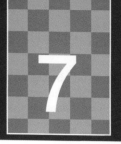
TYPES OF VARIABLES

The data collected from the studies we conduct or critique comprise observations of one or more variables. A variable is a quantity that varies and can take any one of a specified set of values. For example, when collecting information on patient demographics, variables of interest may include gender, race or age. As described by the psychologist Stanley Stevens in 1946, research data usually fall into one of the following four types of variables:

- Nominal
- Ordinal
- Interval
- Ratio

Nominal variable

Variables assessed on a nominal scale are called categorical variables. The order of the categories is meaningless. Examples of nominal variables include:

- Blood type (A, B, AB, O)
- Gender (male, female)
- Surgical outcome (dead, alive)

The categories are mutually exclusive, and simply have names. A special type of nominal variable is a dichotomous variable, which can take only one of two values; for example, gender (male or female). The data collected are therefore binomial. If there are three or more categories for a variable, the data collected are multinomial. For example, for marital status, the categories may be single, married, divorced or widowed. Data collected for nominal variables are usually presented in the form of contingency tables (e.g., 2 × 2 tables).

> **HINTS AND TIPS**
>
> In nominal measurements, the categories of variables differ from one another in name only.

Ordinal variable

An ordinal variable is another type of categorical variable. When a 'rank-ordered' logical relationship exists among the categories, only then is the variable known as an ordinal variable. The categories may be ranked in order of magnitude. For example, there may be ranked categories for disease staging (none, mild, moderate, severe) or for a rating scale for pain, whereby response categories are assigned numbers in the following manner:

- (no pain)
- (mild pain)
- (moderate pain)
- (severe pain)
- (unbearable pain)

The distance or interval between the categories is not known. Referring to our example above, you do not know whether the distance between 1 (no pain) and 2 (mild pain) is the same as the distance between 3 (moderate pain) and 4 (severe pain). It is possible that respondents falling into categories 1, 2 and 3 are actually very similar to each other, while those falling into pain category 4 and 5 are very different from the rest (Fig. 7.1).

> **COMMON PITFALLS**
>
> While a rank order in the categories of an ordinal variable exists, the distance between the categories is not equal.

Interval variable

In addition to having all the characteristics of nominal and ordinal variables, an interval variable is one where the distance (or interval) between any two categories is the same and constant. Examples of interval variables include:

- temperature, i.e., the difference between 80°F and 70°F is the same as the difference between 70°F and 60°F.
- dates, i.e., the difference between the beginning of day 1 and that of day 2 is 24 hours, just as it is between the beginning of day 2 and that of day 3.

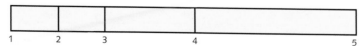

Fig 7.1 Ordinal measurement of pain score.

Interval variables do not have a natural zero point. For example, in the temperature variable, there is no natural zero, so we cannot say that 40°F is twice as warm as 20°F. On some occasions, zero points are chosen arbitrarily.

Ratio variable

In addition to having all the characteristics of interval variables, a ratio variable also has a natural zero point. Examples of ratio variables include:

- height
- weight
- incidence or prevalence of disease

Fig. 7.2 demonstrates the number of children in a family as a ratio scale. We can make the following statements about the ratio scale:

- The distance between any two measurements is the same.
- A family with two children is different from a family with three children (as is true for a nominal variable).
- A family with three children has more children than a family with two children (as is true for an ordinal variable).
- You can say one family has had three more children than another family (as is true for an interval variable).
- You can say one family with six children has had twice as many children as a family with three children (as is true for a ratio variable, which has a true zero point).

TYPES OF DATA

Quantitative (numerical) data

When a variable takes a numerical value, it is either discrete or continuous.

Discrete variable

A variable is discrete if its categories can only take a finite number of whole values. Examples include number of asthma attacks in a month, number of children in a family and number of sexual partners in a month.

Continuous variable

A variable is continuous if its categories can take an infinite number of values. Examples include weight, height and systolic blood pressure.

Qualitative (categorical) data

Nominal and ordinal variables are types of categorical variables, as each individual can only fit into one of a number of distinct categories of the variable. For quantitative variables, the range of numerical values can be subdivided into categories, e.g., column 1 of the table presented in Table 7.1 demonstrates what categories may be used to group weight data. A numerical variable can therefore be turned into a categorical variable. The categories chosen for grouping continuous data should be:

- exhaustive, i.e., the categories cover all the numerical values of the variable.
- exclusive, i.e., there is no overlap between the categories.

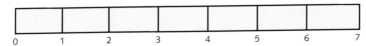

Fig 7.2 Ratio measurement of number of children in a family.

Table 7.1 The frequency distribution of the weights of a sample of medical students				
Weight (kg)	Frequency	Relative frequency (%)	Cumulative frequency	Relative cumulative frequency (%)
40–49.99	1	1.16	1	1.16
50–59.99	3	3.49	4	4.65
60–69.99	11	12.79	15	17.44
70–79.99	20	23.26	35	40.70
80–89.99	30	34.88	65	75.58
90–99.99	15	17.44	80	93.02
100–109.99	6	6.98	86	100.00
TOTAL	86	100.00	86	100.00

DISPLAYING THE DISTRIBUTION OF A SINGLE VARIABLE

Having undertaken a piece of research, producing graphs and charts is a useful way of summarizing the data obtained so they can be read and interpreted with ease. Prior to displaying the data using appropriate charts or graphs, it is important to use frequency distributions to tabulate the data collected.

Frequency distribution

Frequency tables should first be used to display the distribution of a variable. An empirical frequency distribution of a variable summarizes the observed frequency of occurrence of each category. The frequencies are expressed as an absolute number or as a relative frequency (the percentage of the total frequency). Using relative frequencies allows us to compare frequency distributions in two or more groups of individuals. Calculating the running total of the absolute frequencies (or relative frequencies) from lower to higher categories gives us the cumulative frequency (or relative cumulative frequencies; Table 7.1).

HINTS AND TIPS

Frequency tables can be used to display the distribution of:

- nominal categorical variables
- ordinal categorical variables
- some discrete numerical variables
- grouped continuous numerical variables

Displaying frequency distributions

Once the frequencies for your data have been obtained, the next step is to display the data graphically. The type of variable you are trying to display will influence which graph or chart is best suited for your data (Table 7.2).

Bar chart

Frequencies or relative frequencies for categorical variables can be displayed as a bar chart. The length of each bar (either horizontal or vertical) is proportional to the frequency for the category of the variable. There are usually gaps between the bars to indicate that the categories are separate from each other. Bar charts are useful when we want to compare

Table 7.2 Displaying single variables graphically

Type of variable	Display method
Categorical (nominal, ordinal, some discrete)	Bar chart Pie chart
Grouped continuous (interval and ratio)	Histogram

the frequency of each category relative to other categories. It is also possible to present the frequencies or relative frequencies in each category in two (or more) different groups. The grouped bar chart displayed in Fig. 7.3 shows:

- the categories (ethnic groups) along the horizontal axis (x-axis)
- the number of admissions to the cardiology ward (over 1 month) along the vertical axis (y-axis)
- the number of admissions according to ethnic group, which correspond to the length of the vertical bars
- two bars for each ethnic group, which represent gender (male and female)

We can see that most people admitted to the cardiology ward were:

- of male gender (regardless of ethnicity)
- from South Asia (especially Indian in ethnicity)

Alternatively, a stacked bar chart could be used to display the data above (Fig. 7.4). The stacked bars represent the different groups (male and female) on top of each other. The length of the resulting bar shows the combined frequency of the groups.

Pie chart

The frequencies or relative frequencies of a categorical variable can also be displayed graphically using a pie chart. Pie charts are useful for displaying the relative proportions of a few categories. The area of each sector (or category) is proportional to its frequency. The pie chart displayed in Fig. 7.5 shows the various intrinsic factors that were found to cause in-patient falls over one month on a geriatric ward. It is evident that having cognitive impairment was by far the most common intrinsic factor responsible for causing inpatient falls.

HINTS AND TIPS

Pie charts are useful for:

- displaying the relative sizes of the sectors that make up the whole
- providing a visual representation of the data when the categories show some variation in size

---

Histogram

Grouped continuous numerical data are often displayed using a histogram. Although histograms are made up of bars, there are some key differences between bar charts and histograms (Table 7.3). The horizontal axis consists of intervals ordered from lowest to highest. The width of the bars is determined by the width of the categories chosen for the frequency distribution, as shown in Table 7.1. The area of each bar is proportional to the number of cases (frequency) per unit interval. There are no gaps between the bars, as the data represented by the histogram are not only exclusive, but also continuous.

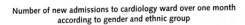

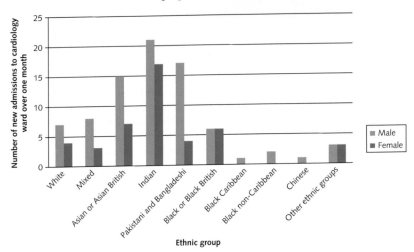

Fig 7.3 Grouped bar chart.

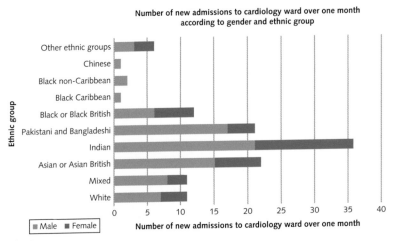

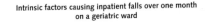

Fig 7.4 Stacked bar chart.

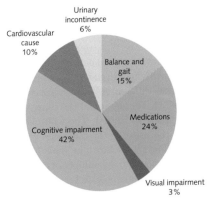

Fig 7.5 Pie chart.

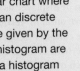

HINTS AND TIPS

Histograms are a special form of bar chart where the data are in continuous rather than discrete categories. Values in a bar chart are given by the length of the bar, while values in a histogram are given by areas. The vertical axis of a histogram does not always show the absolute numbers for each category. An alternative is to show percentages (proportions) on the vertical axis. The length of each bar is the percentage of the total that each category represents. In this case, the total area of all the bars is equal to 100%.

Table 7.3 Bar chart versus histogram

	Bar chart	Histogram
Type of variable displayed	Categorical	Grouped continuous
Purpose	Compare frequencies of each category within a variable	Display the frequency distribution of a variable
Width of bars	Similar	Different
Gap between bars	Yes (however, not strictly true)	No (unless there are no values within a given interval)
What is the frequency represented by?	Length of bar	Area of bar

Example 1

A histogram of the weight data shown in Table 7.1 is presented in Fig. 7.6. As the grouping intervals of the categories are all equal in size, the histogram looks very similar to a corresponding bar chart. However, if one of the categories has a different width than the others, it is important to take this into account:

- If we combine the two highest weight categories, the frequency for this combined group (90–109.99 kg) is 21.
- As the bar area represents frequency, it would be incorrect to draw a bar of height 21 from 90 to 109.99 kg.
- The correct approach would be to halve the total frequency for this combined category, as the group interval is twice as wide as the others.
- The correct height is therefore 10.5, as demonstrated by the dotted line in Fig. 7.6.

Example 2

Fig. 7.7 illustrates the requirement for using areas instead of heights for unequal grouping intervals on the x-axis. Suppose we use a bar chart to display the amount of contrast used during an invasive coronary angiogram, with group intervals organized by 10-mL increments until 100 mL and a final interval of 100 mL to 150 mL (Fig. 7.7A). While a bar chart is quick and easy to plot, the casual reader might think there is a small peak in frequency at the far right of the chart. They need to look closely at the axis labelling to realize that the bars do not cover identical-sized ranges of

contrast volumes. There is a risk of misunderstanding, and indeed an opportunity for deliberate misrepresentation.

A histogram (Fig. 7.7B) is similar to a bar chart, but imposes a requirement that the x-axis is evenly spaced. If you have a block covering a wide range of x values, you must 'spread out' the frequency over a wider horizontal range, so that the height of the bar is not misleadingly large. The correct approach would be to divide the height of the bar by five, as the group interval is five times as wide as the others.

With a bar chart, to interpret the distribution of the data you need to check the x-axis carefully and, if necessary, do some mental arithmetic. With a histogram, one quick look gives you an accurate representation of the distribution.

DISPLAYING THE DISTRIBUTION OF TWO VARIABLES

Selecting an appropriate graph or chart to display the association between two variables depends on the types of variables you are dealing with (Table 7.4).

Numerical versus numerical variables

If both the variables are numerical (or ordinal), the association between them can be illustrated using a scatter plot. When investigating the effect of an exposure on a

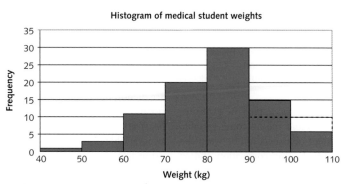

Fig 7.6 Histogram. Please refer to the main text for an explanation for the dotted line.

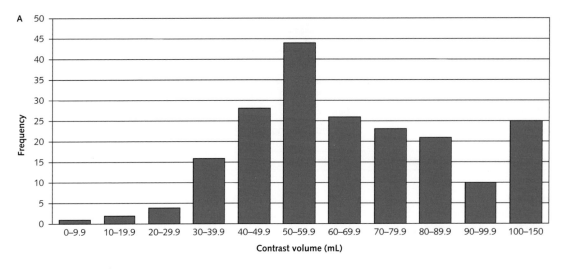

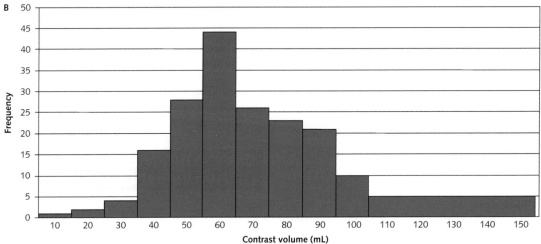

Fig 7.7 Bar chart (A) and histogram distribution (B) of the volume of contrast used during coronary angiography.

Table 7.4 Displaying the association between two variables graphically

Type of variables	Display method
Numerical versus numerical	Scatter plot
Categorical versus categorical	Contingency table
Numerical versus categorical	Box and whisker plot Bar chart Dot plot

particular outcome, it is conventional to plot the exposure variable on the horizontal axis and the outcome variable on the vertical axis. The extent of association between the two variables can be quantified using correlation and/or regression.

Categorical versus categorical variables

If both variables are categorical, a contingency table should be used. Conventionally, the rows should represent the exposure variable, and the columns should represent the outcome variable. Simple contingency tables are 2 × 2 tables where both the exposure and outcome variables are dichotomous. For example, is there an association between smoking status (smoker versus nonsmoker) and heart attacks (heart attack versus no heart attack)? The two variables can be compared and a P-value generated using a chi-squared test or Fisher exact test (discussed in Chapter 20).

Numerical versus categorical variables

Box and whisker plot

A box and whisker plot displays the following information (the numbers underneath correspond to the numbers labelled in Fig. 7.8):

1. The sample maximum (largest observation) – top end of whisker above box
2. The upper quartile – top of box
3. The median – line inside box
4. The lower quartile – bottom of box
5. The sample minimum (smallest observation) – bottom end of whisker below box
6. Which observations, if any, are considered to be outliers

The central 50% of the distribution of the numerical variable is contained within the box. Consequently, 25% of observations lie above the top of the box, and 25% lie below the bottom of the box. The spacings between the different parts of the box indicate the degree of spread and skewness of the data (discussed later).

A box and whisker plot can be used to compare the distribution of a numerical outcome variable in two or more exposure groups, i.e., if comparing two exposure groups, a box and whisker plot would be constructed for each group. For example, if comparing the frequency distribution of haemoglobin level in three separate sample groups (i.e., in smokers, exsmokers and nonsmokers), a separate box and whisker plot would be drawn for each group.

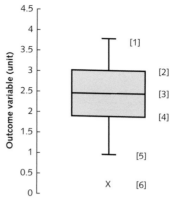

Fig 7.8 Box and whisker plot. Please refer to the main text for a description of the numbering in the square brackets.

> **HINTS AND TIPS**
>
> Other than representing the maximum and minimum sample observations, the ends of the whiskers may signify other measures, such as 1.96 standard deviations above and below the mean of the data. This range (known as the reference interval or reference range) contains the central 95% of the observations. What the whiskers represent should therefore always be defined.

Bar chart

In a bar chart, the horizontal axis represents the different groups being compared, and the vertical axis represents the numerical variable measured for each group. Each bar usually represents the sample mean for that particular group. The bars sometimes have an error bar (extended line) protruding from the end of the bar, which represents either the standard deviation or the standard error of the mean (please refer to Chapter 8 for a discussion on how to interpret errors bars). A bar chart comparing the mean systolic blood pressure between two different groups is presented in Fig. 7.3. Please refer to Table 7.3 for a comparison between histograms and bar charts.

Dot plot

Rather than using a bar to represent the sample mean, each observation can be represented as one dot on a single vertical (or horizontal) line. This is known as an aligned dot plot. However, sometimes there are two or more observations that have the same value. In this situation, a scattered dot plot should be used to ensure that the plotted dots do not overlap (Fig. 7.9). As demonstrated in Fig. 7.9, a summary measure of the data, such as the mean or median, is usually shown on the diagram. In addition to summarizing the data obtained using a graphical display, a frequency distribution can also be summarized using measures of:

- central tendency ('location')
- variability ('spread')

Histograms, box and whisker plots and dot plots are less familiar to most students and junior doctors than bar charts. Table 7.5 summarizes their main advantages and disadvantages.

DESCRIBING THE FREQUENCY DISTRIBUTION: CENTRAL TENDENCY

There are three key measures of central tendency (or location):

- The arithmetic mean
- The mode
- The median

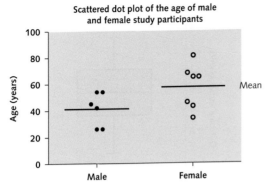

Fig 7.9 Scattered dot plot.

The arithmetic mean

The arithmetic mean is the most commonly used average. 'Mu' (μ) is often used to denote the population mean, while x-bar ($\bar{x}$) refers to the mean of a sample. The mean is calculated by adding up all the values in a set of observations and dividing this sum by the number of values in that set. This description of the mean can be summarized using the following algebraic formula:

$$\bar{x} = \frac{x_1 + x_2 + x_3 + \ldots + x_n}{n}$$

$$\bar{x} = \frac{\sum_{i=1}^{n} x_i}{n}$$

where

- x = variable
- $\bar{x}$ (x-bar) = mean of the variable x
- n = number of observations of the variable
- Σ (sigma) = the sum of the observations of the variable
- Subscripts and superscripts on the Σ = sum of the observations from $i = 1$ to n.

For example, let's look at the raw data of weights from a sample of 86 medical students, ordered from the lowest to the highest value (Fig. 7.10). In this case, as x represents each student's weight, x_1 is the weight of the first individual in the sample and x_i is the weight of the ith individual in the sample:

$$\text{Mean}(x) = \frac{42.34 + 51.56 + 53.54 + \ldots 107.35 + 107.52 + 109.35}{86}$$

$$= 82.3033$$

Therefore, the mean weight of the 86 medical students sampled is 82.3 kg.

The mode

The mode is the most frequently occurring value in a data set. For data that are continuous, the data are usually grouped, and the modal group subsequently calculated. If there is a single mode, the distribution of the data is described as being unimodal. For example, returning to the

Table 7.5 Advantages and disadvantages of bar charts, histograms, box and whisker plots and dot plots

Chart type	Advantages	Disadvantages
Bar charts	– Useful for understanding the distribution from large data sets – Stacked bars can be used to distinguish different levels within the data	– The distribution of the data, the number of data points and their values are all obscured
Histogram	– Visually strong – Good for assessing the shape of the distribution of data with a continuous variable	– Unable to read exact values because data are grouped into categories – The bar widths must be chosen wisely to avoid the shape becoming too compressed or too dispersed – More difficult to compare two or more data sets
Box and whisker plot	– Shows a 5-point summary of the data (minimum, maximum, first quartile, median and third quartile) – Easily compares two or more data sets – Handles extremely large data sets with ease	– Should not be used with small data sets – Not as visually appealing as other graphs – Individual data values are not retained (except for outliers)
Dot plot	– Shows each individual data point – Easy to compare two or more data sets – The distribution of data from multiple categories can easily be compared	– Data that vary widely may be difficult to graph – Not appropriate for representing a large data set because the plot will become cluttered, therefore making it difficult to identify individual data points

Lowest value	66.32	74.23	79.12	83.76	88.24	90.01	98.54
42.34	66.56	74.34	79.43	84.32	88.43	90.43	98.65
51.56	67.33	75.32	79.76	84.87	88.54	91.23	99.35
53.54	68.92	75.43	80.03	85.33	88.65	92.46	99.75
58.49	69.12	75.78	81.23	85.55	88.65	94.56	100.54
60.32	70.33	76.78	81.24	85.63	88.67	95.43	104.23
60.94	71.23	77.65	81.34	85.78	88.75	95.45	106.45
61.44	71.28	77.67	82.34	85.78	89.46	96.45	107.35
62.55	72.35	77.96	82.43	86.43	89.55	96.54	107.52
64.32	73.43	78.45	83.45	87.54	89.64	97.45	109.35
65.87	73.65	78.54	83.45	87.56	89.89	97.46	Highest value

Fig 7.10 Raw data: weights (kg) of a sample of 86 medical students. The numbers are ordered from the lowest to highest value. The two highlighted values are the two middle numbers that are used to calculate the sample median.

data on weights of medical students (Fig. 7.10), which are continuous, the first step in calculating the mode is to group the data as shown in Table 7.1. The modal group is the one associated with the largest frequency. In other words, it is the group with the largest peak when the frequency distribution is displayed using a histogram (Fig. 7.6). In this instance, the modal group is 80 to 89.99 kg. If there is more than one peak, the distribution is called bimodal (for two peaks) or multimodal (for more than two peaks).

The median

The median is the middle value when the data are arranged in ascending order of size, starting with the lowest value and ending with the highest value. If there are an odd number of observations, n, there will be an equal number of values both above and below the median value. This middle value is therefore the $[(n + 1)/2]$th value when the data are arranged in ascending order of size.

If there are an even number of observations, there will be two middle values. In this case, the median is calculated as the arithmetic mean of the two middle values ($[(n/2)]$th and $[(n/2) + 1]$th values) when the data are arranged in ascending order of size. For example, returning to the data on weights of medical students (Fig. 7.10), the sample consists of 86 observations. The median will therefore be the arithmetic mean of the 43rd $[(86/2)]$ and 44th $[(86/2) + 1]$ values when the data are arranged in ascending order of size. These two values are highlighted in the data set (Fig. 7.10). Therefore, the median weight of the 86 medical students sampled is 83.61 kg $[(83.45 + 83.76)/2]$.

DESCRIBING THE FREQUENCY DISTRIBUTION: VARIABILITY

The variability of the data indicates how far the values of a variable in a distribution are spread from the centre of the data.
- There are three key measures of variability (or spread):
  - The range
  - The interquartile range
  - The standard deviation

The range

The range is the difference between the highest and lowest values in the data set. Rather than presenting the actual difference between the two extremes, the highest and lowest values are usually quoted. This is because giving two values provides more information and can be particularly helpful if there is an outlier at one end of the range. For example, returning to the data on weights of medical students (Fig. 7.10), the range is 42.34 to 109.35 kg.

COMMON PITFALLS

Outliers are observations that are numerically different from the main body of the data. While outliers can occur by chance in a distribution, they often indicate that either:
- there was a measurement error, or
- the population has a frequency distribution with a heavy tail (discussed below).

The interquartile range

The interquartile range:
- is the range of values that includes the middle 50% of values when the data are arranged in ascending order of size
- is bounded by the lower and upper quartiles (25% of the values lie below the lower limit and 25% lie above the upper limit)
- is the difference between the upper quartile and the lower quartile

Percentiles

A percentile (or centile) is the value of a variable below which a certain percent of observations fall. For example, the median (which is the 50th centile) is the value below which 50 percent of the observations may be found. The median and quartiles are both examples of percentiles. Although the median, upper quartile and lower quartile are the most common percentiles that we use in practice, any centile can in fact be calculated from continuous data. A particular centile can be calculated using the formula $q(n + 1)$, where q is a decimal between 0 and 1, and n is the number of values in the data set. For example, returning to the data on weights of medical students, which consists of 86 observations (Table 7.4):
- the calculation for the lower quartile is $0.25 \times (86 + 1) = 21.75$; therefore, the 25th centile lies between the 21st and 22nd values when the data are arranged in ascending order of size.
- the 21st value is 73.65 and the 22nd value is 74.23; therefore, the lower quartile is 74.085:

$$73.65 + \left[\left(74.23 - 73.65 \right) \times 0.75 \right] = 74.085.$$

The standard deviation

Population standard deviation

The standard deviation (denoted by the Greek letter sigma, σ) is a measure of the spread (or scatter) of observations about the mean. The standard deviation is the square root of the variance, which is based on the extent to which each observation deviates from the arithmetic mean value. The deviations are squared to remove the effect of their sign, i.e., negative or positive deviations. The mean of these squared deviations is known as the variance. This description of the population variance (usually denoted by σ^2) can be summarized using the following algebraic formula:

$$\sigma^2 = \frac{\Sigma \left(x_i - \bar{x} \right)^2}{n}$$

where
- σ^2 = population variance
- x = variable

- $\bar{x}$ = mean of the variable x
- x_i = individual observation
- n = number of observations of the variable
- Σ = the sum of (the squared differences of the individual observations from the mean)
- The population standard deviation is equal to the square root of the population variance:

$$\sigma = \sqrt{\sigma^2}$$

Sample standard deviation

When we have data for the entire population, the variance is equal to the sum of the squared deviations, divided by n (number of observations of the variable). When handling data from a sample, the divisor for the formula is $(n - 1)$ rather than n. The formula for the sample variance (usually denoted by s^2) is:

$$S^2 = \frac{\Sigma \left(x_i - \bar{x} \right)^2}{n-1}$$

The sample standard deviation is equal to the square root of the sample variance:

$$S = \sqrt{S^2}$$

For example, returning to the data on weights of medical students (Fig. 7.10), the variance is:

$$S^2 = \frac{\left(42.34 - 82.303 \right)^2 + \left(51.56 - 82.303 \right)^2 + \ldots + \left(109.35 - 82.303 \right)^2}{86-1}$$

$$= \frac{15252.123}{85} = 179.437 \, \text{kg}^2$$

The standard deviation is:

$$S = \sqrt{179.437} = 13.395 \text{kg}$$

As the standard deviation has the same units as the original data, it is easier to interpret than the variance.

THEORETICAL DISTRIBUTIONS

Probability distributions

Earlier in this chapter we explained that the observed data of a variable can be expressed in the form of an empirical frequency distribution. When the empirical distribution of our data is approximately the same as a particular probability distribution (which is described by a mathematical model), we can use our theoretical knowledge of that probability distribution to answer questions about our data. These questions usually involve evaluating probabilities.

The rules of probability

A probability measures the chance of an event occurring. It is described by a numerical measure that lies between 0 and 1:

- If an event has a probability of 0, it cannot occur.
- If an event has a probability of 1, it must occur.

Mutually exclusive events

If two events (A and B) are mutually exclusive (both events cannot happen at the same time), then the probability of event A happening OR the probability of event B happening is equal to the sum of their probabilities.

$$\text{Probability}(A \text{ and } B) = P(A) + P(B)$$

For example, Table 7.6 shows the probabilities of the range of grades achievable for Paper 1 on 'Study Design' and Paper 2 on 'Statistical Techniques' for the Evidence-Based Medicine exam. The probability of a student passing Paper 1 is $(0.60 + 0.20 + 0.10) = 0.90$.

Independent events

If two events (A and B) are independent (the occurrence of one event makes it neither ore nor less probable that the other occurs), then the probability of both events A AND B occurring is equal to the product of their respective probabilities:

$$\text{Probability}(A \text{ and } B) = P(A) \times P(B)$$

For example, referring to Table 7.6, the probability of a student passing both Paper 1 and Paper 2 is:

$$\left[\left(0.60 + 0.20 + 0.10\right) \times \left(0.50 + 0.25 + 0.05\right)\right]$$
$$= 0.90 \times 0.80 = 0.72$$

Defining probability distributions

If the values of a random variable are mutually exclusive, the probabilities of all the possible values of the variable can be illustrated using a probability distribution. Probability distributions are theoretical and can be expressed mathematically. Each type of distribution is characterized by certain parameters such as the mean and the variance. In order to make inferences about our data, we must first determine whether the mean and variance of the frequency distribution of our data correspond to the mean and variance of a particular probability distribution. The probability distribution is based on either continuous or discrete random variables.

Continuous probability distributions

As the data are continuous, there are an infinite number of values of the random variable x. Consequently, we can only derive probabilities corresponding to a certain range of values of the random variable. If the horizontal x-axis represents the range of values of x, the equation of the distribution can be plotted. The resulting curve resembles an empirical frequency distribution, and is known as the probability density function. The area under the curve represents the probabilities of all possible values of x, and those probabilities (which represent the total area under the curve) always summate to 1.

Applying the rules of probability described previously, the probability that a value of x lies between two limits is equal to the sum of the probabilities of all the values between these limits. In other words, the probability is equal to the area under the curve between the two limits (Fig. 7.11). The following distributions are based on continuous random variables.

The normal (Gaussian) distribution

In practice, the normal distribution is the most commonly used probability distribution in medical statistics. It is also referred to as the Gaussian distribution or as a bell-shaped curve. The probability density function of the normal distribution:

- is defined by two key parameters: the mean (μ) and the variance (σ^2)
- is symmetrical about the mean and is bell-shaped (unimodal; Fig. 7.12A)
- shifts to the left if the mean decreases (μ_1) and shifts to the right if the mean increases (μ_2), provided that the variance (σ^2) (and therefore the standard deviation) remains constant (Fig. 7.12B)

Table 7.6 Probabilities of grades for the Evidence-Based Medicine exam

	Paper 1 (study design)	Paper 2 (statistical techniques)
Fail	0.10	0.20
Pass	0.60	0.50
Pass with merit	0.20	0.25
Pass with distinction	0.10	0.05
Total probability	1	1

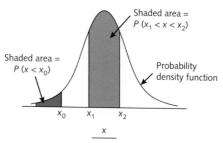

Fig 7.11 The probability density function of a variable (x).

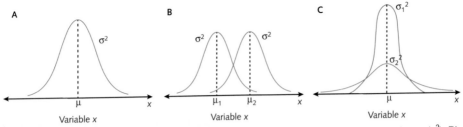

Fig 7.12 Shifting the probability density function of a variable (*x*) by varying the mean (μ) or the variance (σ²). Please refer to the main text for a full description of the three panels.

- becomes more peaked (curve is tall and narrow) as the variance decreases (σ_1^2) and flattens (curve is short and wide) as the variance increases (σ_2^2), provided that the mean (μ) remains fixed (Fig. 7.12C).

The mean, median and mode of the distribution are identical and define the location of the curve.

COMMON PITFALLS

It is worth noting that there is no relation between the term 'normal' used in a statistical context and that used in a clinical context.

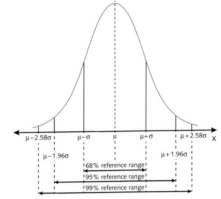

Fig 7.13 Reference range.

Reference range

We can use the mean and standard deviation of the normal distribution to determine what proportion of the data lies between two particular values. For a normally distributed random variable *x* with mean μ and standard deviation σ:

- 68% of the values of *x* lie within one standard deviation of the mean (μ – σ to μ + σ). In other words, the probability that a normally distributed random variable lies between (μ – σ) and (μ + σ) is 0.68.
- 95% of the values of *x* lie within 1.96 standard deviations of the mean (μ – 1.96σ to μ + 1.96σ). In other words, the probability that a normally distributed random variable lies between (μ – 1.96σ) and (μ + 1.96σ) is 0.95.
- 99% of the values of *x* lie within 2.58 standard deviations of the mean (μ – 2.58σ to μ + 2.58σ). In other words, the probability that a normally distributed random variable lies between (μ – 2.58σ) and (μ + 2.58σ) is 0.99.

These intervals can be used to define an additional measure of spread in a set of observations: the reference range. For example, if the data are normally distributed, the 95% reference range is defined as follows: (μ – 1.96σ) to (μ + 1.96σ); 95% of the data lies within the 95% reference range (Fig. 7.13). The 68% and 99% reference ranges can be defined using a similar approach. Considering the normal distribution is symmetrical, we can also say that:

- 16% of the values of *x* lie above (μ + σ), and 16% of the values of *x* lie below (μ – σ)
- 2.5% of the values of *x* lie above (μ + 1.96σ), and 2.5% of the values of *x* lie below (μ – 1.96σ)
- 0.5% of the values of *x* lie above (μ + 2.58σ), and 0.5% of the values of *x* lie below (μ – 2.58σ).

'Standard' normal distribution

As you may be thinking, there are an infinite number of normal distributions depending on the values of the mean and the standard deviation. A normal distribution can be transformed (or standardized) to make a 'standard' normal distribution, which has a mean of 0 and a variance of 1. The standard normal distribution allows us to compare distributions and perform statistical tests on our data.

Other continuous probability distributions

On some occasions, the normal distribution may not be the most appropriate distribution to use for your data.

- The chi-squared distribution is used for analysing categorical data.
- The t-distribution is used under similar circumstances as those for the normal distribution, but when the

sample size is small and the population standard deviation is unknown. If the sample size is large enough ($n > 30$), the t-distribution has a shape similar to that of the standard normal distribution.

- The F-distribution is the distribution of the ratio of two estimates of variance. It is used to compare probability values in the analysis of variance (ANOVA; discussed in Chapter 20).

Discrete probability distributions

As the data are discrete, we can derive probabilities corresponding to every possible value of the random variable x. The sum of the probabilities of all possible mutually exclusive events is 1. The main discrete probability distributions used in medical statistics are as follows:

- The Poisson distribution is used when the variable is a count of the number of random events that occur independently in space or time, at an average rate, i.e., the number of new cases of a disease in the population.
- The binomial distribution is used when there are only two outcomes, e.g., having a particular disease or not having the disease.

Skewed distributions

A frequency distribution is not always symmetrical about the mean. It may be markedly skewed with a long tail to the right (positively skewed) or the left (negatively skewed).

Positively skewed distributions

For positively skewed distributions (Fig. 7.14A), e.g., the F-distribution:

- the mass of the distribution is concentrated on the left
- there is a long tail to the right
- the mode is lower than the median, which in turn is lower than the mean (mode < median < mean)

Negatively skewed distributions

For negatively skewed distributions (Fig. 7.14B):

- the mass of the distribution is concentrated on the right
- there is a long tail to the left
- the mean is lower than the median, which in turn is lower than the mode (mean < median < mode)

TRANSFORMATIONS

If the observations of a variable are not normally distributed, it is often possible to transform the values so that the transformed data are approximately normal. Transforming the values to create a normal distribution is beneficial, as it allows you to use statistical tests based on the normal distribution (discussed in Chapter 20). When a transformation is used, all analyses, including calculating the mean or 95% confidence interval (discussed in Chapter 8), should be carried out on the transformed data. However, the results are back-transformed into their original units when interpreting the estimates. Note: P-values (discussed in Chapter 8) are not back-transformed.

The logarithmic transformation

The logarithmic transformation:

- is the most common choice of transformation used in medical statistics
- is used where continuous data are not normally distributed and are highly skewed to the right
- stretches the lower end of the original scale and compresses the upper end, thus making positively skewed data more symmetrical (Fig. 7.14C)

Log-transformed variables are said to have a lognormal distribution. When log transforming data, we can choose to take logs to any base, but the most commonly used are base 10 ($\log_{10} y$, the 'common' log) base e ($\log_e y = \ln y$, the 'natural' log). Following log transformation of the data, calculations are carried out on the log scale. For example, we can calculate the mean using log-transformed data.

The geometric mean

The mean calculated using log-transformed data is known as the geometric mean. For example, let's look at a few values from the data set of 500 triglyceride level measurements, which have a positively skewed distribution (Table 7.7). The triglyceride level values are first log-transformed to the base e. The mean of all 500 transformed values is:

$$= \frac{\begin{array}{c} 0.2624 + 0.4055 + (-0.9163) + \\ 0.8329 + (-0.5108) + \ldots + 1.4586 \end{array}}{500}$$

$$= \frac{177.4283}{500} = 0.3549$$

The geometric mean is the antilog of the mean of the log-transformed data:

$$= \exp(0.3549) = e^{0.3549} = 1.43 \text{mM}$$

Similarly, in order to derive the confidence interval for the geometric mean, all calculations are performed on the log scale, and the two limits are back-transformed at the end.

It is impossible to log transform negative values, and the log of 0 is −∞. If there are negative values in your data, it is possible to add a small constant to each value prior to transforming the data. Following back-transformation of your results, this constant needs to be subtracted from the final value. For example, if you add 4 units to each value prior to log transforming your data, you must remember to subtract 4 units from the calculated geometric mean.

Calculating the antilog

As any base can be used to log-transform your data, it is important that you understand some basic rules when working with logs.

Rule 1: Don't worry … It's actually quite easy!

Rule 2: You can log transform your value using the formula:

$$\log a^x = y$$

where

- a = the 'base'
- x = the value you are transforming
- y = the result of the transformation

Rule 3: You can back-transform (antilog) your result, y, using the formula:

$$a^y = x$$

For example, if $\log_e 4 = \ln 4 = 1.3863$, then $e^{1.3863} = 4$.

The square transformation

The square transformation is used where continuous data are not normally distributed and are highly skewed to the left. It achieves the reverse of the log transformation. Referring to Fig. 7.14B, if the variable y is skewed to the left, the distribution of y^2 is often approximately normal (Fig. 7.14D).

Table 7.7 Logarithmic transformation of positively skewed data

Measurement	Triglyceride level (mM)	$\log_e$(triglyceride level)
1	1.3	0.2624
2	1.5	0.4055
3	0.4	-0.9163
4	2.3	0.8329
5	0.6	-0.5108
...	...	...
500	4.3	1.4586

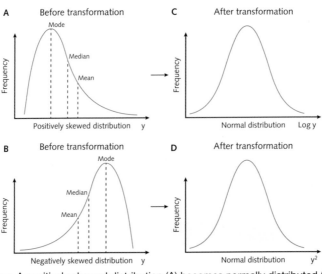

Fig 7.14 Skewed distribution. A positively skewed distribution (A) becomes normally distributed (C) following a logarithmic transformation. A negatively skewed distribution (B) becomes normally distributed (D) following a square transformation.

CHOOSING THE CORRECT SUMMARY MEASURE

The measure used to describe the centre and spread of the distribution of your data depends on the type of variable you are dealing with (Fig. 7.15). In addition to the information summarized in Fig. 7.15, there are three key points:

- A frequency distribution can be used for all four types of variables: nominal, ordinal, interval and ratio.
- As previously discussed, a positively skewed distribution can sometimes be transformed to follow a normal distribution. In this situation, the central tendency is usually described using the geometric mean. However, the standard deviation cannot be back-transformed correctly. In this case, the untransformed standard deviation or another measure of spread, such as the interquartile range, can be given.
- For continuous data with a skewed distribution, the median, range and/or quartiles are used to describe the data. However, if the analyses planned are based on using means, it would be sensible to give the standard deviations. Furthermore, the use of the reference range holds even for skewed data.

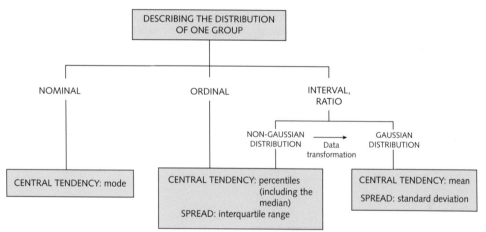

Fig 7.15 Choosing the correct summary measure.

● **Chapter Summary**

- A categorical variable is for mutually exclusive, but not ordered, categories.
- An ordinal variable is one where the order matters but not the difference between values.
- An interval variable is a measurement where the difference between two values is meaningful.
- A ratio variable has all the properties of an interval variable and also has a clear definition of 0.
- A variable is discrete if its categories can only take a finite number of whole values and continuous if its categories can take an infinite number of values.
- Nominal and ordinal variables are types of categorical variables, as each individual data point can only fit into one of a number of distinct categories of the variable.
- Frequency tables can be used to display the distribution of nominal categorical variables, ordinal categorical variables, some discrete numerical variables and grouped continuous numerical variables.
- Frequencies or relative frequencies for categorical variables can be displayed as a bar chart or a pie chart.
- Grouped continuous numerical data are often displayed using a histogram.

- Selecting an appropriate graph or chart to display the association between two variables depends on the types of variables you are dealing with (numerical versus numerical: scatter plot; categorical versus categorical: contingency table; numerical versus categorical: box and whisker plot, bar chart or dot plot).
- The arithmetic mean is calculated by adding up all the values in a set of observations and dividing the sum by the number of values in that set.
- The mode is the most frequently occurring value in a data set.
- The median is the middle value when the data are arranged in ascending order, starting with the lowest value and ending with the highest value.
- The range is the difference between the highest and lowest values in the data set.
- The interquartile range is the range of values that includes the middle 50% of values when the data are arranged in ascending order.
- The standard deviation (denoted by the Greek letter sigma, s) is a measure of the spread (or scatter) of observations about the mean.
- The normal distribution is the most commonly used probability distribution in medical statistics. It is also referred to as the Gaussian distribution or as a bell-shaped curve. The mean, median and mode of the distribution are identical and define the location of the curve.
- For positively skewed distributions, the mass of the distribution is concentrated on the left, and there is a long tail to the right (the mode is lower than the median, which in turn is lower than the mean).
- For negatively skewed distributions, the mass of the distribution is concentrated on the right, and there is a long tail to the left (the mean is lower than the median, which in turn is lower than the mode).

FURTHER READING

Bland, M., 2015. An Introduction to Medical Statistics, second ed. Oxford University Press, Oxford.

Kirkwood, B.R., Sterne, J.A.C., 2003. Essential Medical Statistics, second ed. Blackwell Publishing, Oxford.

Motulsky, H.J. GraphPad Statistics Guide. Available from: https://www.graphpad.com/guides/prism/7/statistics/index.htm [Accessed 21st September 2018].

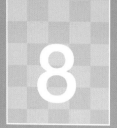
HYPOTHESIS TESTING

As described in Chapter 2, the aim of a study may involve examining the association between an 'intervention' or 'exposure' and an 'outcome'. We must first state a specific hypothesis for a potential association.

The null and alternative hypotheses

A hypothesis test uses sample data to assess the degree of evidence that there is against a hypothesis about a population. We must always define two mutually exclusive hypotheses:

- Null hypothesis (H_0): there is no difference/association between the two variables in the population
- Alternative hypothesis (H_A): there is a difference/ association between the two variables in the population

For example, we may test the null hypothesis that there is no association between an exposure and outcome. In 1988, the Physicians' Health Study Research Group reported the results of a 5-year trial to determine whether taking aspirin reduces the risk of a heart attack. Patients had been randomly assigned to either aspirin or a placebo. The hypotheses for this study can be stated as follows:

- Null hypothesis (H_0): There is no association between taking aspirin and the risk of a heart attack in the population. This is equivalent to saying:

$$H_0 : \left(\text{risk of heart attack in group treated with aspirin} \right) - \left(\text{risk of heart attack in group treated with placebo} \right) = 0$$

- Alternative hypothesis (H_A): There is an association between taking aspirin and the risk of a heart attack in the population. The difference in the risk of a heart attack between the aspirin and placebo groups does not equal 0.

Having defined the hypotheses, an appropriate statistical test is used to compute the P-value from the sample data. The P-value provides a measure of the evidence for or against the null hypothesis. If the P-value shows evidence against the null hypothesis being tested, then the alternative hypothesis must be true.

CHOOSING A SAMPLE

The basic principle of statistics is simple: using limited amounts of data (your 'sample'), we wish to make the strongest possible conclusions about the wider population. For these conclusions to be valid, we must consider the precision and accuracy of the analyses.

Accuracy versus precision

Distinguishing between accuracy and precision is an important but difficult concept to understand. Imagine playing darts. The bull's-eye in the centre of the dartboard represents the population statistic we are trying to estimate, and each dart represents a statistic calculated from a study sample. If we throw nine darts at the dartboard, we see one of four patterns regarding the accuracy and precision of the sample estimates (darts) relative to the population statistic (bull's-eye) (Fig. 8.1).

Accuracy

The study sample is accurate if it is representative of the population from which it was chosen (Fig. 8.1A and B). This can be achieved if:

- each individual in the population has an equal chance of being selected (random sampling)
- the selection is completely independent of individual characteristics such as age, sex or ethnic origin

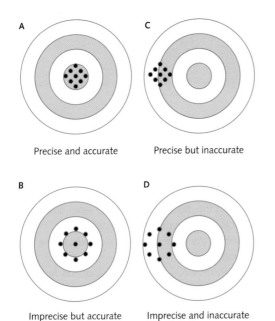

Precise and accurate   Precise but inaccurate

Imprecise but accurate   Imprecise and inaccurate

Fig. 8.1 Precision versus accuracy. (A) Precise and accurate. (B) Precise but inaccurate. (C) Imprecise but accurate. (D) Imprecise and inaccurate.

The methods used in practice to ensure randomisation are discussed in Chapter 11. If samples were not randomly selected (systematic bias), any sample estimate, on average, will differ from the population statistic. As a result, the study sample will be inaccurate (Fig. 8.1C and D).

Precision
The amount of variation between the sample estimates determines the precision of the study sample.

If there is little variability between the sample estimates, i.e., the estimates themselves are similar to each other, the study sample statistics are more precise (Fig. 8.1A and C). The less precise the sample statistics (Fig. 8.1B and D), the less we are able to narrow down the likely values of the population statistic.

COMMON PITFALLS

When choosing between accurate and precise study samples, it is more important to be accurate, because, on average, the study sample estimates will be closer to the true population value.

EXTRAPOLATING FROM SAMPLE TO POPULATION

Having chosen an appropriate study sample, the rules of probability are applied to make inferences about the overall population from which the sample was drawn (Fig. 8.2). The following steps are used:

- Choose a random sample from population.
- Take a measurement for each subject, denoted as x.
- Calculate the mean value of the sample data, denoted as x.
- As estimates vary from sample to sample, calculate the standard error and the confidence interval (CI) of the mean to take this imprecision into account.

Standard error of the mean

When we choose only one sample for a study, the sample mean will not necessarily be the same as the true population mean. Due to sampling variation, different samples selected from the same population will give different sample means. Therefore, if we calculate the mean from all the possible samples in the population, we would have a distribution of the sample mean. This distribution has the following properties:

- If the sample is large enough, the sampling distribution of the mean will follow a Gaussian distribution (even if the population is not Gaussian!), because of the central limit

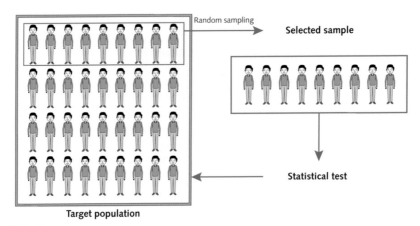

Random sampling → Selected sample

Statistical test

Target population

Fig. 8.2 Hypothesis testing.

THE *P*-VALUE

Statistical hypothesis testing

In the previous section we used CIs to make statistical inferences about the size of the difference in the incidence risk of first stroke between individuals randomized to either simvastatin or a placebo. Simvastatin lowered the 5-year incidence risk of stroke by 1.4% (95% CI 0.8% to 2.0%). However, observing different proportions between the simvastatin and placebo groups is not enough to convince you to conclude that the populations have different proportions. It is possible that the two populations (simvastatin and placebo) have the same proportion (i.e., simvastatin does not lower the 5-year incidence risk of stroke) and that the difference observed between the sample proportions occurred only by chance. To find out whether the apparent difference you observed could easily have arisen through the play of chance, without any true difference, you need to use the rules of probability to calculate a *P*-value.

As discussed in the 'Hypothesis testing' section at the start of this chapter, there are four basic steps involved in hypothesis testing. The first step is to specify the hypothesis and the alternative hypothesis:

- Null hypothesis (H_0): There is no association between simvastatin and the risk of stroke in individuals with a high risk of cardiovascular disease.
- Alternative hypothesis (H_A): There is an association between simvastatin and the risk of stroke in individuals with a high risk of cardiovascular disease.

The second step is to collect the data (Table 8.3) and determine what statistical test is appropriate for data analysis (discussed in Chapter 20). As we are comparing nominal data in two unpaired groups, with $n > 5$ in each cell (Table 8.3), the statistical test most appropriate for analysing these data is the chi-squared test (please refer to Fig. 20.3). The final two steps are to calculate and then interpret the *P*-value.

Calculating the *P*-value

The *P*-value:

- is calculated using a statistical test that tests the null hypothesis
- is derived from the test statistic, which is dependent on the standard error of the difference between means or proportions
- is a probability, with a value ranging between 0 and 1
- represents the weight of evidence there is for or against the null hypothesis

Specifically, the *P*-value is the probability that the difference between the two groups would be as big or bigger than that observed in the current study if the null hypothesis was true. A total of 0.05 or 5% is traditionally used as the cut-off.

- If the observed *P*-value is less than 0.05 ($P < 0.05$), there is good evidence that the null hypothesis is not true. This is related to the type I error rate (discussed later in this chapter).
- $P < 0.05$ is described as statistically significant.
- $P \geq 0.05$ is described as not statistically significant.

For example, let's assume that you compared two means and obtained a *P*-value of 0.02. This means:

- there is a 2% chance of observing a difference between the two groups at least as large as that observed even if the null hypothesis is true (i.e., even if the two population means are identical)
- random sampling from similar populations would lead to a smaller difference between the two groups than that observed on 98% of occasions, and at least as large as that observed on 2% of occasions

One-tail versus two-tail *P*-values

When comparing two groups, you will either calculate a one-tail or two-tail *P*-value. Both types of *P*-values are based on the same null hypothesis. The two-tail *P*-value answers the following question: assuming that the null hypothesis is true, what is the chance that random samples from the same population would have means (or proportions) at least as far apart as those observed in the current study, with either group having the larger mean (or proportion)? For example, using the chi-squared test for our data on simvastatin and stroke risk, the two-tail *P*-value was calculated. With a two-tail *P*-value of < 0.0001, we have extremely significant evidence against the null hypothesis.

The one-tail *P*-value answers the following question: assuming that the null hypothesis is true, what is the chance that random samples from the same population would have means (or proportions) at least as far apart as observed in the current study, with the specified group having the larger mean (or proportion)? A one-tail *P*-value is used when we can predict which group will have the larger mean (or proportion), even prior to collecting any data. Common sense or prior data may inform us that a potential difference can only go in one direction. Therefore, if the other group ends up with the larger mean (or proportion), we should attribute that outcome to chance, even if the difference is relatively large. If you are unsure whether to choose a one-tail or two-ail *P*-value, it is advisable to choose the latter.

STATISTICAL SIGNIFICANCE AND CLINICAL SIGNIFICANCE

The aim of this section is to highlight that:

- a statistically significant result does not necessarily imply that the differences observed are clinically significant
- a non–statistically significant result does not necessarily imply that the differences observed are clinically insignificant, merely that the differences may have occurred due to chance

Inferences about the target population can be made from the sample using the 95% CI and the *P*-value (Fig. 8.4). Considering both *P*-values and CIs are derived from the size of the difference in means (or proportions) between two groups and the standard error of this difference, the two measures are closely related.

Interpreting small *P*-values (*P* < 0.05)

If the *P*-value is small (*P* < 0.05), the difference observed is unlikely to be due to chance. As previously discussed, a small *P*-value suggests we have evidence against the null hypothesis, i.e., there truly is a difference. However, you must consider whether this difference is large enough to be clinically significant. Therefore, based on scientific judgement, statistical significance may not equate to clinical significance.

Using confidence intervals

When comparing two means, the 95% CI will not contain 0 if the *P*-value is less than 0.05. It is important to interpret the clinical significance of both ends of the CI of the difference between means. For example,

- The CI may include differences that are all considered to be clinically significant. In this case, even the lower end of the CI represents a difference that is large enough to be clinically important.
- The CI may only include differences that are relatively small and insignificant. In other words, even though the 95% CI does not include a difference of 0 (remember, the *P*-value is < 0.05), the treatment effect is too small to be considered clinically significant. Therefore, the treatment has an effect, but a relatively small one.
- Sometimes you're stuck in the middle! The CI may range from a clinically unimportant difference to one that is considered clinically significant. Even though

you can be 95% confident that the true difference is not 0, you cannot reach a solid conclusion.

Interpreting large *P*-values (*P* ≥ 0.05)

If the *P*-value is large (*P* ≥ 0.05), the difference observed may be due to random sampling. As previously discussed, a large *P*-value suggests that there is not enough evidence against the null hypothesis, i.e., the true means do not differ. This does not imply that the true means are the same. If the true means were equal, finding a difference between the means as large as the one observed in the current study would be due to chance.

Using confidence intervals

When comparing two means, the 95% CI will range from a negative number to a positive number if the *P*-value is less than 0.05. It is important to interpret the clinical significance of both ends of the CI of the difference between means. For example,

- The CI may range from a negative number, which has no clinical importance, to a positive number that actually has clinical significance. In this case, with 95% confidence, the difference in means is either 0, small and unimportant or large enough to be clinically significant. No solid conclusion can be made. You would reach the same conclusion even if both ends of the CI included clinically significant differences.
- The CI may only include differences that are relatively small and insignificant. Therefore, with 95% confidence, the difference in means is either 0 or small enough to be considered clinically unimportant. In conclusion, the results seem to confirm the negative findings.

P-values and study design

On some occasions, due to poor study design, e.g., having a small sample size, you may calculate a *P*-value that should be interpreted with caution. For example, a potentially clinically significant difference may be observed in a small study; however, the *P*-value is ≥ 0.05. Therefore, the results are statistically nonsignificant. Such a scenario can be avoided if statistical power is considered during the design phase of a study.

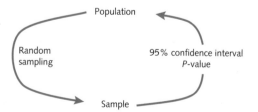

Fig. 8.4 Extrapolating from sample to population using statistical methods.

STATISTICAL POWER

Type I and type II errors

When we test a hypothesis, we make a conclusion about whether an effect is statistically significant (or not). However, when we decide to either reject or fail to reject the null hypothesis, due to random sampling, our decision can be wrong in two ways. We can:

- incorrectly reject the null hypothesis when it is true (type I error)
- incorrectly fail to reject the null hypothesis when it is false (type II error)

Type I error

When random sampling causes your data to show a statistically significant association/difference, but there really is no effect, a type I error has been made. Your conclusion that the sample means of the two groups are really associated/different is incorrect. Type I error is also the alpha (α) level in our hypothesis test, which represents the level of error we are willing to accept in our study.

Type II error

When random sampling causes your data to not show a statistically significant association/difference, but there really is an effect, a type II error has been made. Your conclusion that the sample means of the two groups are not really associated/different is incorrect. The letter beta (β) is used to represent type II error. The different types of error are summarized in Table 8.7.

Definitions of power and β

Due to the statistical nature of hypothesis testing, statistical error must always be considered when making a conclusion about whether an effect is statistically significant. For example, even though a treatment is known to have an effect on the measured variable, a statistically significant difference might not be obtained in your study. Due to chance, your sample data may yield a P-value greater than your predefined cut-off for α (most commonly 0.05, as discussed above). Let's illustrate this point by looking at a study investigating the effect of amitopril, a new (made-up) angiotensin-converting enzyme inhibitor (ACEi; anti-hypertensive drug), on systolic blood pressure.

Statistical power: the effect of amitopril on systolic blood pressure

A hypothetical phase II clinical trial (clinical trial phases are discussed in Chapter 10) has shown that amitopril, taken at a dose of 10 mg daily for 12 weeks, can reduce the systolic blood pressure by more than ramipril, the gold standard ACEi used in clinical practice. Considering that one tablet of amitopril costs a staggering eight times as much as one tablet of ramipril, a cost-effectiveness analysis (discussed in Chapter 21) was carried out. Based on this economic review, the Department of Health issued a statement saying that amitopril could only be approved for use in clinical practice if it reduced the systolic blood pressure by more than 30 mmHg compared to the reduction in systolic blood pressure caused by ramipril.

Table 8.7 Hypothesis testing outcomes

		Null hypothesis	
		True	False
Null hypothesis test decision	Reject	*Type I error* False positive Alpha (α)	*Correct outcome* True positive Power (1 – β)
	Fail to reject	*Correct outcome* True negative (1 - α)	*Type II error* False negative Beta (β)

You decide to carry out a phase III clinical trial by randomizing young, nonsmoking, white males, with newly diagnosed hypertension, to either amitopril or ramipril for 12 weeks, measuring the systolic blood pressure before and after treatment. Taking the above into account, let's specify the null and alternative hypotheses:

- The null hypothesis (H_0): the mean change in systolic blood pressure caused by amitopril minus the mean change in systolic blood pressure caused by ramipril is ≤30 mmHg
- The alternative hypothesis (H_A): the mean change in systolic blood pressure caused by amitopril minus the mean change in systolic blood pressure caused by ramipril is >30 mmHg

The sampling distributions for the null and alternative hypotheses are presented in Fig. 8.5. We sample 5000 patients and compare our sample mean to the null hypothesis. Referring to Fig. 8.5, the sample mean from our study has been plotted on the null hypothesis sampling distribution. With α set at 0.05, our mean of 36.2 mmHg falls within our rejection region, so we can reject the null hypothesis. As shown on the graph, the probability that our study will yield a nonstatistically significant result is defined by β. Correctly rejecting a false null hypothesis is therefore represented by the (1 – β) area of the distribution. Remember that the area under the curve represents the probability or relative frequency. We can therefore calculate the statistical power by calculating the probability that our sample mean falls into the (1 – β) area under the distribution curve. If we perform many similar studies with the same sample size, we can deduce the following:

- due to chance, some studies will yield a statistically significant finding with a P-value less than α
- in other studies, the mean change in systolic blood pressure caused by amitopril minus the mean change in systolic blood pressure caused by ramipril will be less than 30 mmHg, and will not be statistically significant

If there is a high chance that our study will yield a statistically significant result, the study design has high power. As amitopril really causes a difference in blood pressure, the probability that our study will yield a not–statistically significant result is defined by β, which represents type II error,

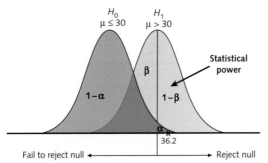

Fig. 8.5 Statistical power. Please refer to the main text for a detailed explanation.

as discussed above. β is therefore equal to 1.0 minus power (or 100% minus power (%)).

HINTS AND TIPS

Even if there is a real numerical difference between group means, a statistically significant difference will not always be found in every study. The power of the study predicts the fraction of studies that are expected to yield a *P*-value that is statistically significant.

Interpreting nonsignificant results

If your results fail to show a statistically significant association/difference, we can use CIs and power analyses to interpret the negative data. These approaches allow two different ways of analysing the data using the same assumptions.

Confidence interval

The CI (discussed above) approach shows how precisely you have determined the differences of interest. It combines the variability (SD) and sample size to generate a CI for the population mean. Having calculated the CI, it is up to you to put the result in a scientific context.

Power analysis

A power analysis can assist you in putting your results in perspective. This approach helps you plan or criticize other similar studies. Having failed to reject the null hypothesis, statistical power calculations firstly involve estimating a value for the sample mean for the alternative hypothesis. We usually estimate this value from previously published studies on the same topic or from a small pilot study. Having established this value, you then ask what is the probability that a study (with the same sample size) would have resulted in a statistically significant difference if your alternative hypothesis was true.

HINTS AND TIPS

The statistical power should be addressed:
1. when we fail to reject the null hypothesis
2. when we are planning a study

To demonstrate the steps involved in interpreting non-significant results, let's look at a study investigating whether alterations of receptor numbers can affect the force of contraction in chronic heart failure.

Confidence interval versus power analysis: receptor numbers in chronic heart failure

Catecholamines such as noradrenaline have positive inotropic effects on the human heart via their effect on β_1- and β_2-adrenergic receptor binding. Despite having identified other receptor systems in the heart that also mediate these positive inotropic effects, the cardiac β-adrenergic receptor pathway is the most powerful mechanism for influencing cardiac contractility.

Since nearly all β-adrenergic cardiac receptors are required to induce maximal inotropic effects on the heart, any reduction in the number of β-adrenergic receptors will consequently lead to a reduced inotropic response to receptor stimulation. Due to the enhanced sympathetic drive to the heart in chronic heart failure, there are reasons to believe that β-adrenergic receptors are reduced in these patients. Theoretical results are shown in Table 8.8.

Assuming that the values follow a Gaussian distribution, an unpaired *t*-test (see Fig. 20.2) was used to compare the means of the two unmatched groups. The mean receptor number per heart cell was very similar in the two patient groups, and the *t*-test yielded a very high *P*-value. We can therefore conclude that the cardiac cells of people with chronic heart failure do not have an altered number of β-adrenergic receptors. Let's use the CI of the difference in mean receptor number between the groups and also carry out a power analysis to assist us in interpreting the results.

Table 8.8 Receptor numbers per cardiac cell

Variable	Chronic heart failure	Control
Number of subjects	20	19
Mean β-adrenergic receptor number per cardiac cell	143	137
Standard deviation	33.8	58.2

Using confidence intervals

The difference in mean receptor number between the two groups is six receptors per cardiac cell. The 95% CI for the difference between the group means = −25 to 37 receptors/cardiac cell. Therefore, the true increase in mean receptor number per cardiac cell in subjects with chronic heart failure is six receptors/cell (95% CI −25 to 37). We can be 95% sure that this interval contains the true difference between the mean receptor number in the two subject groups. If the average number of β-adrenergic receptors per cardiac cell is 140, the CI includes possibilities of an 18% decrease or a 26% increase in receptor number. In other words, there could be a relatively big increase/decrease or no change in receptor number in people with chronic heart failure.

To put this into a scientific perspective, as the majority of β-adrenergic receptors in the normal human heart are needed to cause a maximal inotropic effect, an 18% decrease in receptor number seems scientifically important. On the other hand, the 26% increase in receptor number is biologically trivial, as even in the normal human heart there are still a few spare receptors when maximal inotropic effects have been reached.

Using power analysis

If there truly is a change in cardiac β-adrenergic receptor number in people with chronic heart failure, what was the power of the study to find this change? This depends on how large the difference in mean receptor number between normal and chronic heart failure subjects actually is. This is denoted by the term delta, as shown in the power curve in Fig. 8.6. Considering that the majority of β-adrenergic receptors in the normal human heart are needed to cause a maximal inotropic effect, any decrease in receptor number is biologically significant. For this reason, even if the difference in the number of receptors was only 10%, we would want to conduct follow-up studies. As the mean number of receptors per cardiac cell is 140, we would want to find a difference of approximately 14 receptors per cell (delta = 14). Reading this value off the power curve below, we can conclude that the power of this study to find a difference of 16 receptors per cardiac cell was only about 15%. In other words, even if the difference really was this large, this study had only a 15% chance of finding a statistically significant result. With such low power to detect a biologically significant finding, we are unable to make any confident conclusions from the study results.

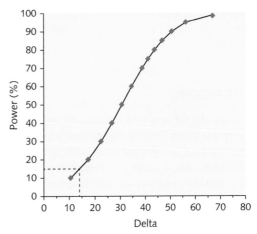

Fig. 8.6 The power curve. For this particular power curve, a delta of 14 was associated with a study power of 15%. Please refer to the main text for a detailed description.

Sample size calculations

When comparing means or proportions between two groups in a study, it is important to choose a sample size that gives a high probability of detecting a given effect size (if it exists). Power analysis can be used to calculate the sample size we need for a future study using the following information:

- The power of the test (1 − β): More subjects will be needed if a higher power is chosen.
- The significance level (α): More subjects will be needed if a smaller significance level is chosen.
- The SD: More subjects will be needed if the data have a high SD. The SD is estimated from previous data or pilot studies. If different SDs are expected in the two groups, the average is used.
- The minimum difference (d) that is clinically important: More subjects will be needed if you want to detect a smaller difference.
- The value for K: This is a multiplier that depends on the significance level and the power of the study, and is derived from the normal distribution. Table 8.9 shows common values of K used for studies comparing two proportions or two means.

Table 8.9 Multipliers (K) for studies comparing two proportions or two means

Power (1 − β)	Significance level (α)		
	0.05	0.01	0.001
80%	7.8	11.7	17.1
90%	10.5	14.9	20.9
95%	13.0	17.8	24.3
99%	18.4	24.1	31.6

The number of subjects required in each group depends on whether we are comparing two means or two proportions (Table 8.10).

Determining acceptable statistical power levels

How much power is required?
Referring to the power graph in Fig. 8.6, the rate of increase in power starts to reduce dramatically at around 80% as we increase the power of the study further. Several investigators therefore choose a sample size to obtain an 80% power in their study. As power is equal to $(1 - \beta)$, your choice of an acceptable level of power for your study should ideally be influenced by the consequences of making a type II error.

How to get more power?
There are four main factors that influence statistical power:

- The significance level
- The sample size
- The effect size
- One-tail versus two-tail tests

The significance level
Referring to Fig. 8.7A, we can see that there is a direct relationship between:

- our significance level (α), which is our type I error
- β, which is our type II error
- the statistical power $(1 - \beta)$

When we increase the significance level α, we decrease β and increase the statistical power of the study $(1 - \beta)$ to find a real difference (Fig. 8.7B). However, this approach also increases the chance of falsely finding a 'significant' difference.

The sample size
The sample size also has a direct influence on the level of statistical power. When we increase the sample size, we get a more accurate estimate for the population parameter. In other words, the SD of the sampling distribution (standard error) is smaller. The distributions for the null and alternative hypotheses therefore become more leptokurtic, with a more acute peak around the mean and thinner, longer tails. This decreases our type II error (β) and increases the statistical power of the study (Fig. 8.7C).

The effect size
The degree of distance between the alternative hypothesis and null hypothesis distributions denotes the effect size. We estimate the anticipated difference between the alternative and null hypotheses from the literature. The larger the effect size, the smaller the type II error (β) and, consequently, the larger the statistical power $(1 - \beta)$ (Fig. 8.7D). Understandably, the investigator has no control over the effect size. All studies have higher power to detect a large difference between groups than to detect a small one.

One-tail versus two-tail tests
One-tail (directional) tests have more power than two-tail (nondirectional) tests. This topic has been discussed earlier in this chapter.

Table 8.10 Sample size calculations using power analysis

(i) Sample size – comparing two means	(ii) Sample size – comparing two proportions
$n = \dfrac{2K\left(SD^2\right)}{d^2}$	$n = \dfrac{K\left[P_1\left(1-P_1\right) + P_2\left(1-P_2\right)\right]}{\left(P_1 - P_2\right)}$

d, The minimum clinically important difference; K, a multiplier calculated from the power $(1 - \beta)$ and the significance level (α); P1, the expected population proportion in group A; P2, the expected population proportion in group B; SD, the standard deviation expected.

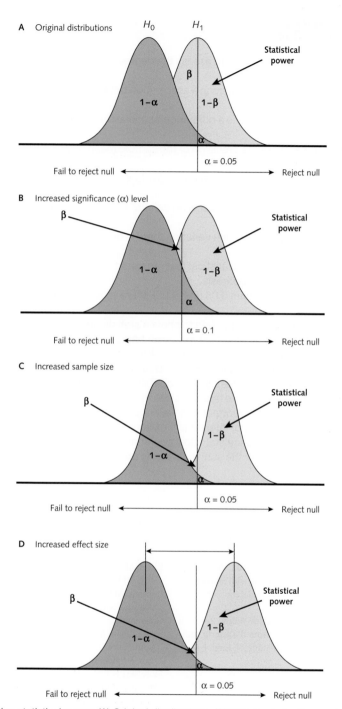

Fig. 8.7 Factors influencing statistical power. (A) Original distributions. (B) Increased significance (α) level. (C) Increased sample size. (D) Increased effect size. Please refer to the main text for additional details.

● **Chapter Summary**

- A hypothesis test uses sample data to assess the degree of evidence that there is against a hypothesis about a population.
- Null hypothesis (H0): there is no difference/association between the two variables in the population.
- Alternative hypothesis (HA): there is a difference/association between the two variables in the population.
- The standard error measures the precision of the sample mean as an estimate of the population mean.
- The standard deviation informs us how far an individual observation is likely to be from the true population mean.
- The confidence interval shows how precise an estimate the sample mean is of the true population mean.
- The reference range shows how much variation there is between the individual observations in the sample.
- The P-value is calculated using a statistical test representing the weight of evidence that there is for or against the null hypothesis.
- If the observed P-value is less than 0.05 ($P < 0.05$), there is good evidence that the null hypothesis is not true.
- When random sampling causes your data to show a statistically significant association/difference, but there really is no effect, a type I error has been made.
- When random sampling causes your data to not show a statistically significant association/difference, but there really is an effect, a type II error has been made.
- The power of a binary hypothesis test is the probability that the test correctly rejects the null hypothesis when the alternative hypothesis is true.
- When conducting a study, it is important to have enough statistical power to have a high likelihood of capturing the effect of interest (if it exists).
- The four main factors that influence statistical power are the significance level, the sample size, the effect size and whether the statistical test is one-tail or two-tail.

REFERENCES

Heart Protection Study Collaborative Group, 2002. MRC/BHF Heart Protection Study of cholesterol lowering with simvastatin in 20 536 high-risk individuals: a randomised placebo-controlled trial. Lancet 360, 7–22.

Steering Committee of the Physicians' Health Study Research Group, 1988. Preliminary report: findings from the aspirin component of the ongoing Physicians' Health Study. N. Engl. J. Med. 318, 262–264.

FURTHER READING

Bland, M., 2015. An Introduction to Medical Statistics, second ed. Oxford University Press, Oxford.

Columb, M.O., Atkinson, M.S., 2016. Statistical analysis: sample size and power estimations. BJA Education 16 (5), 159–161.

Greenland, S., Senn, S.J., Rothman, K.J., Carlin, J.B., Poole, C., Goodman, S.N., Altman, D.G., 2016. Statistical tests, P values, confidence intervals, and power: a guide to misinterpretations. Eur. J. Epidemiol. 31, 337–350.

Motulsky, H.J. GraphPad Statistics Guide. Available from: https://www.graphpad.com/guides/prism/7/statistics/index.htm [Accessed 21st September 2018].

Sensitivity analysis

A sensitivity analysis determines whether the findings of the meta-analysis are robust to the methodology used to obtain them. This analysis involves comparing the results of two or more meta-analyses, which are calculated using different assumptions. These assumptions may include:

- omitting low quality studies
- omitting studies with questionable eligibility for the systematic review
- omitting studies that appear to be outliers
- omitting a particular trial that you feel is driving the result, i.e., the largest trial.
- using several alternative imputed values where there are missing data for one of the trials; this may be an issue when including cluster-randomized trials or cross-over trials

HINTS AND TIPS

A sensitivity analysis may involve carrying out a meta-analysis with and without an assumption and subsequently comparing the two results to determine whether there is a statistically significant difference between them.

PRESENTING META-ANALYSES

The results of meta-analyses are often presented in a standard way known as a 'forest plot' (Fig. 9.1). In a forest plot:

- the individual study results are represented by a circle or a square to indicate the study estimate
- the size of the circle or square is proportional to the weight for that individual study in the meta-analysis
- the horizontal line running through the circle or square corresponds to the 95% confidence interval for that particular study estimate
- the centre of the diamond (and broken vertical line) represents the summary effect estimate of the meta-analysis
- the 95% confidence interval for the summary effect estimate corresponds to the width of the diamond
- the unbroken vertical line is at the null value (1)
- the studies are often displayed in chronological order

EVALUATING META-ANALYSES

Interpreting the results

If the confidence interval of the summary effect estimate (width of diamond) crosses the null value (solid vertical

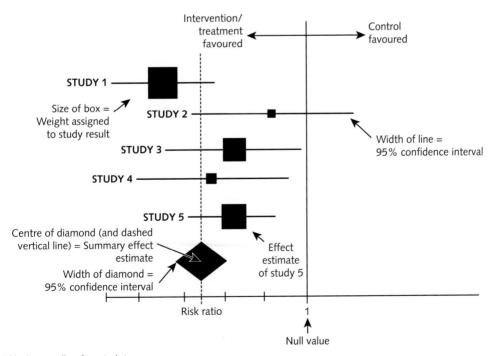

Fig. 9.1 Understanding forest plots.

line), this is equivalent to saying that there is no statistically significant difference in the effects in the exposure and control groups. When interpreting the results, it is important to consider the following questions:

- Is there strong evidence for an exposure effect?
- Is there unexplained variation in the exposure effect across individual studies?
- Are the results applicable to your patient?
- Are there any implications for future research?
- Are there any potential sources of bias?

Bias in meta-analyses

Production of evidence

It is crucial that threats to the internal validity of a study (confounding, bias and causality) are reviewed for all studies included in the systematic review. The three main threats to internal validity are discussed in turn for each of the key study designs in their respective chapters. Methodological checklists for critically appraising the key study designs covered in this book are provided in Chapter 22.

Dissemination of evidence

While systematic reviews aim to include all high quality studies that address the review question, finding all relevant studies may not be possible. Failure to include all relevant studies in a meta-analysis may lead to the exposure effect being under- or overestimated.

The analyses reported in a published article are more likely to show a statistically significant difference between the competing groups than they are to show a nonsignificant difference. All outcomes should be included in the final research report so as to avoid outcome-reporting bias. In general, studies with significant, positive results are more likely to be:

- considered worthy of publication (publication bias)
- published in English (language bias)
- published quickly (time lag bias)
- published in more than one journal (multiple publication bias)
- cited in subsequent journals (citation bias)

Reporting bias incorporates all of these types of bias. The overrepresentation in systematic reviews of studies with positive findings may lead to reviews being biased towards a positive exposure effect.

Publication bias

Detecting publication bias

Publication bias in meta-analyses is usually explored graphically using 'funnel plots'. These are scatter plots with the following features:

- The relative measure of exposure effect (risk ratio or odds ratio) is depicted on the horizontal axis. The exposure effects are usually plotted on a logarithmic scale to ensure that effects of the same magnitude but in opposite directions, such as odds ratios of 0.3 and 3, are equidistant from the null value.
- The standard error of the exposure effect (which represents the study size) is depicted on the vertical axis.

As the sample size of a study increases, there is an increase in the precision (and a reduction in the standard error) of the study in being able to estimate the underlying exposure effect. Furthermore, we would expect more precise studies (with larger sample sizes) to be less affected by the play of chance. In summary:

- large studies have more precision (i.e., low standard error), and the exposure estimates are expected to be closer to the pooled estimate
- small studies have less precision (i.e., high standard error), and the exposure estimates are expected to be more variable (more widely scattered) about the pooled estimate

In the absence of publication bias, the plot will resemble a symmetrical inverted funnel (Fig. 9.2A). If there is publication bias, where smaller studies showing no statistically significant effect remain unpublished, the funnel plot will have an asymmetrical appearance with the lower righthand (or lefthand, depending on the research question) corner of the plot missing (Fig. 9.2B). As demonstrated in Fig. 9.2B, publication bias will lead to an overestimation of the treatment effect (the risk ratio has decreased from 0.7 to approximately 0.5).

Other causes of funnel plot asymmetry

Publication bias is not the only cause of funnel plot asymmetry. Smaller studies may produce more extreme treatment effects. If these studies have poorer methodological quality, which may happen if they are not carefully designed, they may be more vulnerable to overstating the benefit observed from an exposure/treatment. Common examples of this are when the physician delivering treatment or recording

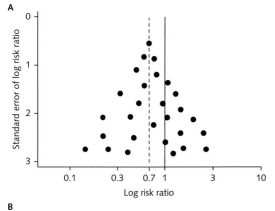

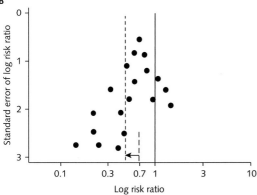

Fig. 9.2 Understanding funnel plots. Please refer to the main text for a full description.

journals will not consider trials for publication unless they are registered from the start. It has also been suggested that journals should consider studies for publication based only on the literature review and study methodology. The reviewers are therefore 'blind' to the actual results of the study. Importantly, a study should have sufficient power to detect a clinically significant effect (if one exists); therefore, trials that have a small sample size (and therefore a low power to detect an exposure effect) should be discouraged.

outcome measurements is unblinded. Critical appraisal of the methodological quality of all study types is discussed in their respective chapters. Sometimes asymmetry cannot be assessed, as there are too few studies. As a rule of thumb, tests for funnel plot asymmetry should not be used when there are fewer than ten studies in the meta-analysis, as the test power will usually be too low to distinguish real asymmetry from chance.

HINTS AND TIPS

Funnel plots should be used to identify whether there is a tendency for smaller studies in a meta-analysis to have larger exposure effect estimates. In other words, funnel plots indicate whether 'small study effects' are present.

Preventing publication bias

One solution has been to put all ongoing established trials on a register that is openly available to everyone, such as ClinicalTrials.gov, a registry of clinical trials run by the United States National Library of Medicine. Some

Advantages of systematic reviews:

- Appear at the top of the 'hierarchy of evidence' that informs evidence-based practice, thus giving us the best possible estimate of any true effect.
- Can shorten the time lag between research practice and the implementation of new findings in clinical practice.
- Are relatively quicker and less costly to perform than a new study.
- Critically appraise and synthesize large amounts of information in order to reduce errors (including bias) and improve the accuracy and reliability of the findings.
- Provide results that, compared to a single study, can often be generalized to a broader population across a wider range of settings.
- Provide evidence that the phenomenon is robust and transferable, if the studies included in the review give consistent results.
- Indicate any sources of variation can be studied if the studies included in the review give inconsistent results
- Have high power to detect exposure effects and estimate these effects with greater precision than single studies, if meta-analysis is also performed.

Disadvantages of systematic reviews

- Require considerably more effort than traditional reviews.
- Pose clinical questions that are often too narrow, thus reducing the applicability of the findings to your patient.
- Sometimes review interventions that do not reflect current practice.

- May not be possible to perform if there is an insufficient number of high-quality studies available for review.
- Do not consider the underlying physiological effects of an intervention.
- Rarely consider the fact that some interventions are delivered as part of a larger package of care.

KEY EXAMPLE OF A META-ANALYSIS

In 1995, Joseph Lau and his colleagues performed a meta-analysis of controlled trials assessing the effects of prophylactic antibiotics on mortality rates following colorectal surgery, i.e., the perioperative mortality. There were 21 trials carried out between 1969 and 1987 that compared the effect of an antibiotic prophylaxis regimen on perioperative mortality rates after colorectal surgery. The meta-analysis of these trials is presented in Fig. 9.3A as a forest plot:

- The odds ratio and 95% confidence intervals are shown on a logarithmic scale, with the pooled treatment effect estimate at the bottom of the forest plot.
- Compared to an inactive treatment, antibiotic prophylaxis was shown to reduce the number of perioperative deaths following colorectal surgery in 17 of the 21 trials, i.e., the odds ratio was less than the null value (1) in 17 trials.
- However, none of these 17 trials had a statistically significant finding, i.e., the 95% confidence interval of the treatment effect estimate crossed the null value (1) in all 17 trials.
- Despite this, the pooled treatment effect odds ratio estimate of all 21 trials was in favour of using antibiotic prophylaxis to reduce the number of perioperative deaths following colorectal surgery, i.e., the P value was < 0.05.

If a new meta-analysis had been performed each time the results of a new trial were reported, would we have realized the beneficial effects of antibiotic prophylaxis prior to 1987 (when the 21st trial was published)? The answer is clear from the cumulative meta-analysis presented in Fig. 9.3B:

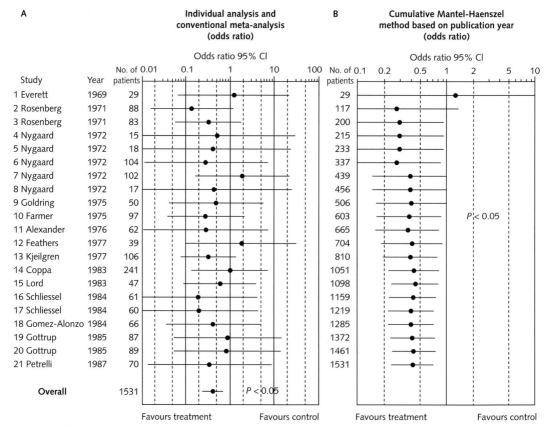

Fig. 9.3 (A) Conventional and (B) cumulative meta-analyses of 21 trials on the effect of prophylactic antibiotics on perioperative mortality rates following colorectal surgery. CI, confidence interval. (Reproduced with permission from Lau J, et al. *J Clin Epidemiol* 1995;48:45–57.)

Randomized controlled trials

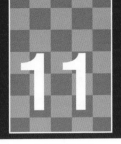

11

A methodological checklist for the critical appraisal of randomized controlled trials is provided in Chapter 22.

WHY CHOOSE AN INTERVENTIONAL STUDY DESIGN?

As introduced in Chapter 10, interventional studies test whether intervening in some way leads to a measurable variation in the outcome. The intervention usually involves a particular treatment or practice. As highlighted by Hennekens (1987), interventional studies test either preventative or therapeutic interventions, including:

- prophylactic agents
- therapeutic agents
- surgical procedures
- diagnostic agents
- health service strategies

Therapeutic trials are conducted on individuals with a particular disease to evaluate whether a certain procedure or agent has an effect on a specific outcome, such as symptomatic relief or reduced mortality.

Preventative trials are conducted to investigate whether a certain procedure or agent reduces the risk of developing a particular disease. The individuals (or entire communities) enrolled at the beginning of the trial should be free from that disease, but deemed to be at risk.

Regardless of whether the trial is based on therapeutic or preventative research:

- the intervention being tested is allocated (not always randomly) by the investigator to a group of participants (the test group).
- the study participants are followed to compare the test group to the control group (gold standard treatment, placebo or no treatment).

Let us start by discussing one of the most commonly used interventional study designs—the parallel randomized controlled trial (RCT).

PARALLEL RANDOMIZED CONTROLLED TRIAL

Study design

An RCT is an interventional study during which study participants are allocated randomly to different treatment options. This process of randomization makes RCTs the most rigorous method for determining a cause–effect relationship between an intervention and an outcome, thus placing RCTs at the top of the hierarchy of evidence (Chapter 2: Fig. 2.2). This method is improved when the results of several RCTs are pooled together in a meta-analysis as part of a systematic review (discussed in Chapter 9).

A 'parallel' RCT involves randomly assigning individuals from the sample population to different interventions (usually two: the intervention and control 'arm', e.g., gold standard treatment or placebo, but there may be more than two arms). These groups are then followed to assess the effectiveness of the intervention compared with the control. This parallel study design is illustrated in Fig. 11.1. The essential steps involved in a parallel RCT are:

- Formulate the hypothesis (discussed in Chapter 2). For example, we hypothesize that the 2-year mortality risk in patients receiving treatment A is 30% lower than the mortality risk in patients receiving standard treatment.
- Define the methods of recruitment, including the *inclusion* and *exclusion criteria*.
- Define the intervention (discussed earlier).
- Define the comparison group.
- Determine the sample size.
- Specify the outcome measures that will be used to assess the effectiveness of the intervention.
- Obtain ethical approval.
- Obtain informed consent before the study participants are randomized to either the intervention or control.
- Generate and conceal an allocation sequence to ensure randomization.
- Indicate whether the assessors and/or study participants ha ve any knowledge of the treatment allocation (blinding).
- Perform an intention to treat (ITT) analysis.

Inclusion/exclusion criteria

There should be a clear statement highlighting which individuals are eligible to participate in the RCT. Some individuals are excluded if it is too risky (contraindicated) to give them the new intervention or to deny them the conventional (gold standard) treatment. Some investigators restrict eligibility:

- if they feel the intervention will have a different effect on different groups of people. Therefore, to ensure the internal validity of the findings, patients with multiple comorbid conditions are often excluded.

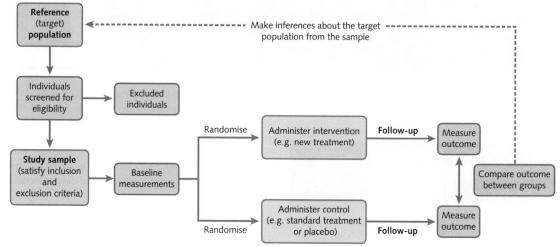

Fig. 11.1 Parallel randomized controlled trial design.

- by focusing on patients with a higher event rate, which:
  - lowers the required sample size (by increasing the power of the study).
  - shortens the required follow-up period.

Having strict inclusion or exclusion criteria limits the generalizability and thus the external validity of the RCT. If the inclusion or exclusion criteria are too restrictive, the results of the study can only be applied to a select group of patients. However, these trials provide data that are often used to inform the justification of the intervention for all patients. The resulting guidelines may therefore offer a simplistic, potentially inadequate approach to using the intervention in clinical practice.

Members of the population may be excluded if they have certain comorbid conditions or have particular demographic features (race, age, gender etc.). For example, trials on the treatment of hypertension were, for decades, limited to patients under 80 years old. There was therefore no evidence on which to base a decision on treating hypertension in older patients. As a result, the myth that hypertension in the elderly did not require treatment was allowed to persist, at the expense of the lives of many older patients!

EXCLUDING PATIENTS WITH COMORBID CONDITIONS

The question of excluding patients with comorbidities, such as those with cardiac, pulmonary or renal disease, is complex. These patients are more likely to die from or to become ill with conditions unrelated to the intervention

being tested, therefore weakening the power of the trial to detect a real benefit from the intervention. Having never been tested in those with comorbidities (often elderly patients), the intervention may perform unpredictably in these patients when used in clinical practice.

HINTS AND TIPS

The patient groups commonly under-represented in trials include:

- pregnant women
- children
- individuals with comorbidities
- the elderly
- individuals with mental illness, including dementia

Choice of comparator

An important feature of an RCT is that it should be comparative. Once you have defined the intervention, the next step is to choose the comparator. The intervention and comparison groups are known as the 'arms' of the trial. There may be more than one comparison group, e.g., comparing the intervention to the gold standard treatment (best available treatment) and a placebo. The comparator chosen (known as the control) will influence how we interpret the evidence about the intervention from the trial. If the control chosen is an inert treatment (placebo), the intervention may show a more favourable outcome (i.e., the importance of the new intervention may be overstated) than if the control was another active treatment, such as the gold standard. Placebos or using no treatment at all are known as negative controls. Using the gold standard treatment is known as a positive control.

As highlighted by the Declaration of Helsinki, item 32, comparing the active intervention against a placebo when an active treatment exists would be unethical:

- The benefits, risks, burdens and effectiveness of a new intervention must be tested against those of the best current proven intervention, except in the following circumstances:
  - The use of placebo or no treatment is acceptable in studies where no current proven intervention exists.
  - Where for compelling and scientifically sound methodological reasons the use of placebo is necessary to determine the efficacy or safety of an intervention and the patients who receive placebo or no treatment will not be subject to any risk of serious or irreversible harm.

HINTS AND TIPS

A placebo is a treatment that looks, feels and even tastes like the new interventional drug being tested but contains no active ingredients whatsoever.

Sample size

The RCT should have enough subjects to detect the smallest difference in effect size between the two study arms that is considered clinically important. This effect size should be informed by clinical judgement, not by the effect sizes observed in previous studies. A larger sample size is required if the clinically significant difference in effect size is small. In other words, more data are required to distinguish a small treatment effect from a random sampling error.

In addition to the effect size, the size of the sample is dependent on:

- the power of the study (often set at 80% or 90%)
- the stated level of statistical significance (often $P = 0.05$)
- the standard deviation of the data for each group.

Please refer to Chapter 8, Statistical power, for a discussion on how to calculate the sample size for a comparative study. If the sample size has not been given in a research paper or if the calculated sample size was not achieved, the study may have been too small to detect a clinically significant difference in effect size between the two groups.

The outcome measure

The outcome is what is measured in all subjects after they have been treated with the intervention or control. The outcome measured as part of the trial should give the investigator an indication of the effectiveness of the intervention (and the control). Various aspects of the outcome need to be considered for a proper assessment of the effectiveness of the treatment:

- Disease aspect: Mortality or survival rate, lab tests, complications, major events, side effects, etc.
- Patient aspect: Health-related quality of life, symptoms, activities of daily living, etc.
- Economic aspect: Service utilization (e.g., length of stay or number of GP visits) or social disruption (e.g., returning to work).
- The outcome measured should be:
- precisely defined to reduce or to prevent misclassification
- measureable
- repeatable
- reliable
- relevant from both a healthcare professional and patient point of view.

It is important to specify how and at what time points these outcomes should be measured. While many outcome measures may be assessed in a single trial, it is important to define a primary outcome variable, which:

- is the outcome of greatest importance.
- has the strongest influence on the conclusions of the trial.
- will inform the sample size calculations.

Data on secondary outcomes are used to evaluate any additional effects caused by the intervention. While the sample size may be large enough to determine a treatment effect based on the primary outcome, it may be too small to detect a clinically important difference on secondary outcomes.

Ethical issues

All research studies must receive research ethics committee approval before being undertaken. Considering that the investigators are 'intervening' in people's lives, RCTs raise a number of important ethical issues, including:

- Clinical equipoise
- Informed consent.

Clinical equipoise

Healthcare professionals treating the patients must have sufficient doubt about the relative effectiveness of the treatments being compared. There must be no evidence that the new intervention is better, worse or the same as any of the treatments currently being used in clinical practice or the placebo. As highlighted earlier in this chapter, if an effective treatment is available, the new intervention should be compared against it and not against a placebo. If these criteria are satisfied, the trial has 'clinical equipoise'.

Informed consent

Informed consent must be obtained from all patients recruited to an RCT. Two key steps must be addressed to ensure that an individual gives valid informed consent to participate in a trial:

- Disclosure of information
- Capacity of the subject.

Disclosure requires the investigator to supply the subject with an adequate amount of information so that he or she can make an autonomous decision about whether to participate in the trial. The investigator should use lay language to communicate the details of the study to the eligible subjects. According to the Declaration of Helsinki, item 24:

- Each potential subject must be adequately informed of the aims, methods, sources of funding, any possible conflicts of interest, institutional affiliations of the researcher, the anticipated benefits and potential risks of the study and the discomfort it may entail and any other relevant aspects of the study.

The next step is to ensure that the patient has the capacity to make a decision about participating in the trial. The potential subject must understand the information provided, weigh up the risks and benefits of taking part in the trial and then communicate his or her decision to the investigator. The consent must be voluntary, i.e., the decision made is not subject to external pressure such as coercion or manipulation. Ideally, the consent should be confirmed in writing. However, if this is not possible, it is important to ensure that nonwritten consent is formally documented and witnessed. There is usually a 'cooling-off period' to allow subjects sufficient time to change their minds if they wish to do so. Whether or not the individual decides to participate in the trial, his or her future access to health services or treatment should not be affected.

What if the intervention is perceived by the study participants to be better and more desirable than the control? This may happen if the intervention is a full programme of care, while the control is usual care. For example, in 2009, an RCT assessed the effectiveness of supervised exercise therapy compared with usual care, in patients with patellofemoral pain syndrome. Outcome measures included assessing pain scores, functional status and patient recovery. The intervention group received a standardized exercise programme for 6 weeks and the control group were assigned usual care, which included a 'wait and see'

approach of rest during periods of pain. In trials similar to this, it is not possible to mask the intervention, i.e., the study participants are able to tell which study arm they have been randomly allocated to. In an attempt to prevent subjects from dropping out of the trial if they are allocated to the control group, some investigators decide in advance to offer the new intervention to all subjects randomly allocated to the control group after the end of the trial, assuming the intervention proves to have a beneficial effect. This will have to be taken into account when the trial finances are being considered.

Randomization

Each study participant has the same probability of being allocated to a particular treatment arm. This process is known as random allocation, which forms the essence of RCTs. The purpose of randomization is to balance confounders (both detectable and undetectable) between the study arms of a trial. Randomization ensures that patient characteristics that may affect the outcome measure (potential confounders) are distributed evenly between the study arms of the trial. With this in mind, provided that the trial is reasonably large, any observed differences between the study arms are due to differences in the treatment alone and not due to the effects of confounding factors.

Methods of randomization

There are four main methods used to randomize patients to the different study arms:

- Simple randomization.
- Block randomization.
- Stratified randomization.
- Minimization.

Simple randomization

Random numbers can be generated using a computer program:

- As a patient enters the trial, the computer program provides an allocation code, which refers to a particular treatment.
- An alternative approach is to produce a computer-generated list of sequential random allocations to the different treatment arms.

Block randomization

Because it can take many months before a sufficient number of subjects have been entered into a trial, block randomization is used to ensure that the number of participants assigned to each treatment arm is very similar at any stage during the recruitment process. Computer randomization software can be programmed to ensure that every 'block' of patients (e.g., every hundred) contains an equal number allocated to each arm of the trial. This method is commonly used in smaller trials.

Stratified randomization

Stratified randomization is used to ensure that important baseline confounding factors are more evenly distributed between the treatment arms rather than leaving it to chance. The confounding factors balanced by stratification are usually those that are important prognostic factors for the particular disease you are investigating. For example, in a trial of women with breast cancer, it may be important to have similar numbers of premenopausal and postmenopausal women in each treatment group. Prior to randomization, participants would be separated into two groups (strata) according to their menopausal status. Equal numbers of participants would then be randomly allocated to each treatment arm within the strata. To ensure that there are an equal number of participants in each treatment arm, this method of treatment allocation, within each stratum, may be based on the block randomization method (discussed earlier).

Minimization

Similar to stratified randomization, minimization may be used to balance the numbers of prognostic factors in each treatment arm. In minimization, the first participant is allocated a treatment at random. Each subsequent participant is allocated to the intervention arm that would lead to a better balance between the groups in the variable (prognostic factor) of interest.

> **HINTS AND TIPS**
>
> Patients are not always randomly allocated in equal proportions to the different treatment arms. For example, an investigator may choose a randomization method to ensure that 60% of the study participants receive the intervention while 40% receive the usual treatment. This is still random allocation, as each study participant will have the same 60% probability of being allocated to the intervention. The investigators may wish to obtain extra information about the novel intervention if sufficient information is already known about the effectiveness of the usual treatment.

Allocation sequence concealment

The second part of randomization is to ensure that the random allocation sequence is concealed. This involves making sure that the patients and the investigators enrolling the patients cannot foresee treatment group assignment. If this allocation process is not adequately concealed, there is potential for selection bias and confounding (discussed later). Examples of adequate concealment include:

- central randomization at a site remote from the trial location (usually the gold standard).
- using sequentially numbered, opaque, sealed envelopes (however, this approach is open to tampering).
- coding and packaging drugs at an independent pharmacy in a drug trial.

> **HINTS AND TIPS**
>
> Concealment is different to blinding: while the allocation sequence can always be concealed at the time of recruitment in an RCT, the feasibility of blinding depends on the particular interventions being investigated. Therefore, while all interventions are technically concealable, they are not all blindable!

> **HINTS AND TIPS**
>
> If randomization has been successful, the two treatment arm groups should be similar. The investigators can assess this by measuring and comparing various baseline characteristics, such as age, gender and disease severity, between the two groups. Large differences in the baseline characteristics may be due to:
> - random allocation not being random because of issues with generating or concealing the allocation sequence
> - chance variation, especially if the sample size is small.

Blinding

Blinding refers to patients and investigators (including those involved in recruitment and assessing the outcome) having no knowledge of treatment allocation. Traditionally, blinded RCTs have been classified as 'single-blind', 'double-blind' or 'triple-blind':

- Single-blind: patients have no knowledge of the treatment they will receive.
- Double-blind: both the patient and the study investigators involved in measuring the outcomes of interest have no knowledge of the patient treatment allocation.
- Triple-blind: the patient, the investigators involved in measuring the outcomes of interest and the investigator analysing the data are not aware of the patient treatment allocation.

Due to inconsistencies in the definitions of these terms and lack of clarity in journals, it is better to specify who exactly was blinded and how.

If the intervention is an active drug, it is possible for both the subject and investigator to be blind to treatment allocation if the comparison group takes an inactive placebo, which looks, tastes and feels exactly like the active drug. RCTs may also use an active placebo that mimics the common side effects of the drug under study. For example, in a study assessing the effects of morphine and gabapentin (painkillers) on neuropathic pain, lorazepam was chosen as an active placebo as it mimicked the side-effects of the painkillers (dizziness and sleepiness).

It is important to note that blinding may not be possible if the RCT involves:

- a technology, e.g., surgery versus chemotherapy.
- a programme of care, e.g., exercise therapy versus medication.

In these studies, known as open-label trials, randomization should still be used and the outcome assessor should still be blind (if possible) to which treatment the participant received.

CONFOUNDING, CAUSALITY AND BIAS

Confounding

Confounding occurs when the exposure of interest is not only associated with the risk of disease but also associated with a third variable that provides an alternative explanation for any association measured between the exposure and disease (please refer to Chapter 18 for an in-depth discussion on confounding). As discussed earlier, the aim of random allocation is to ensure that the treatment groups are similar in composition with respect to prognostic factors, demographics or any other factor. In other words, randomizing trial participants reduces confounding between treatment groups. Therefore, any differences in outcome are due to actual differences in the treatment. Confounding would be an issue if, for example, being male was a poor prognostic factor for a given disease and the distribution of sexes was not equal between the treatment groups investigating that disease.

Causality

RCTs are considered the most rigorous of all methods of determining whether a cause–effect relationship exists between an intervention and outcome. As the exposure is assigned at the start of the study, the temporal relationship between exposure and outcome is clear. For a more in-depth discussion on causality, please refer to the Bradford-Hill criteria, which are discussed in Chapter 10.

Bias

The reliability of the results of an RCT also depends on the extent to which potential sources of bias have been avoided. For an introduction to systematic error and bias, please refer to Chapter 12, Bias. Systematic error can be divided into selection bias and measurement bias (Fig. 11.2). As there is

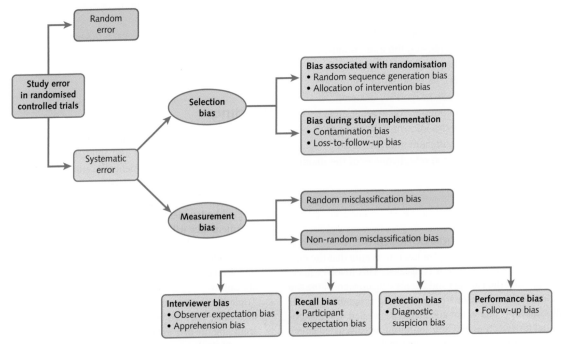

Fig. 11.2 Study error in randomized controlled trials.

usually more interest in showing that an intervention works than in showing that it has no beneficial effect, bias in RCTs tends to lead to an exaggeration in the importance or effectiveness of a new intervention.

Selection bias

Selection bias occurs when the association between an intervention and outcome is different for those who complete the study compared with those who are in the target population. Selection bias may exist when procedures for subject selection or factors that influence subject participation affect the outcome of the study. The main types of selection bias that may occur in RCTs include:

- Bias associated with randomization
  - Random sequence generation bias
  - Allocation of intervention bias.
- Bias during study implementation
  - Contamination bias
  - Loss-to-follow-up bias.

Bias associated with randomization: random sequence generation bias and allocation of intervention bias

If the randomization sequence is not truly random (random sequence generation bias), there is potential for selection bias. Even if the randomization sequence is truly random, selection bias may still be an issue if allocation is not concealed at the time of recruitment (allocation of intervention bias):

- The investigator may recruit patients for the intervention based on their prognosis.
- A patient might decide to take part in the trial only if they are allocated to one treatment arm and not the other.

This will lead to systematic differences between the participants in the different treatment groups. Therefore, differences in the outcome may be explained by preexisting differences between the groups rather than due to differences that exist between the treatments. There is empirical evidence confirming that the effects of new interventions can be exaggerated if an RCT has poor allocation concealment. One study has shown that the intervention effect size may, on average, be exaggerated by as much as 40%.

Bias during study implementation: contamination bias

Contamination may be an issue if there is unintentional (or intentional) application of the intervention in the control group. Alternatively, there may be unintentional (or intentional) failure to give the intervention to those study participants randomly assigned to it. The intervention effect is biased towards the null. Contamination bias occurs more frequently in community RCTs because of the relationships that exist between members who reside in different communities and due to interference from the media or other health professionals. Group randomization (i.e., in cluster randomized trials) reduces the likelihood of contamination bias.

Bias during study implementation: loss-to-follow-up bias

Attrition refers to the loss of subjects during the course of a trial, i.e., these subjects are lost to follow-up. Loss-to-follow-up bias (or attrition bias) refers to systematic differences between the treatment groups in terms of the number of subjects lost or differences in characteristics between those not adhering to the study protocol and those who remain in the study. Attrition applies to those subjects:

- excluded after the allocation process, e.g., if they do not actually satisfy the eligibility criteria.
- who do not adhere to the treatment course (regardless of whether outcome measurements are still taken). If the subject knows which treatment he has been allocated to, this may affect his decision regarding treatment withdrawal or compliance.
- who will not comply with having outcome measurements taken (regardless of whether they adhered to the treatment course).
- who are lost to follow-up for any reason, e.g., they move out of the area or they die when out of the area and their death is not reported to the investigators.

It is important to consider not only why subjects were lost to follow-up but also how many. As already mentioned, it is possible that those subjects lost to follow-up have different characteristics to those who adhere to the trial protocol. The reliability of the results is therefore in question if these two parameters (reason for loss to follow-up and the number of subjects affected) are not comparable between the two treatment groups. For example, participants may drop out due to the side-effects caused by the new intervention. Excluding these participants from the analysis could result in an overestimation of the effectiveness of the intervention, especially when the proportion of people dropping out varies between the treatment groups (thus causing attrition bias). In an attempt to try to minimize the degree of attrition bias, an ITT analysis is usually performed (discussed later).

HINTS AND TIPS

One technique commonly used to assess the likely impact of attrition (loss-to-follow-up) is to calculate the percentage of participants affected. If attrition affects:

- <5% of the study participants, bias will be minimal.
- >20%, then bias is likely to be considerable.

The potential impact of loss to follow-up can be assessed by carrying out a 'best case worst case' sensitivity analysis (discussed later).

Measurement bias

Measurement bias occurs when the information collected for the exposure and/or outcome variables is inaccurate. This type of bias can be divided into random or nonrandom misclassification bias.

Random misclassification bias

Random misclassification bias (also known as nondifferential misclassification bias) can occur when misclassification is the same across the groups being compared. For example, the outcome is equally misclassified in both treatment arms. The treatment groups therefore seem to have more similarities than they actually have, leading to an underestimation (dilution) of the true effect of the intervention on the disease outcome. Random misclassification bias is discussed in further detail in Chapter 12.

Nonrandom misclassification bias

Nonrandom misclassification bias (also known as differential misclassification bias) occurs only when misclassification is different in the treatment groups being compared. It can lead to the intervention effect on the disease outcome being biased in either direction. The main types of nonrandom misclassification bias that may occur in RCTs include:

- Performance bias
  - Follow-up bias
- Detection bias
  - Diagnostic suspicion bias
- Recall bias
  - Participant expectation bias
- Interviewer bias
  - Observer expectation bias
  - Apprehension bias.

Performance bias

Performance bias may exist if the investigators were not kept blind to the treatment allocation. Performance bias is a type of nonrandom misclassification measurement bias. It refers to systematic differences between the two treatment groups in the care that is provided, other than having different treatments. If the investigator knows which treatment arm the patient was allocated to, this may bias the results, either intentionally or unintentionally. Depending on treatment allocation, the investigator might:

- administer other effective interventions (cointerventions)
- perform different investigations
- provide additional advice.

This type of bias is known as follow-up bias. As discussed earlier, there are occasions, however, when blinding is not possible. It is important to think about the likely size and direction of the bias caused by lack of sufficient blinding. Studies have shown that the intervention effect size may be exaggerated by as much as 17%.

Detection bias

Detection bias refers to systematic differences between the groups in how the outcomes are measured. It is a type of nonrandom misclassification measurement bias. Similar to the concept behind performance bias, failure to blind the investigators assessing the outcome can lead to variation in how the outcome is measured between the groups. This is especially the case if the outcomes measured are subjective. In other words, knowledge of the subject's prior exposure status to a putative cause may have an influence on the intensity (and possibly the outcome) of the diagnostic process. This type of detection bias is known as diagnostic suspicion bias.

In addition to ensuring that the outcome assessors are kept blind to treatment allocation (and other important confounding factors), valid and reliable methods should be used to determine precisely defined outcomes in all subjects. It is also important that an RCT has an appropriate length of follow-up to identify the outcome of interest. For example, for outcomes that occur late following an exposure, an RCT with a relatively short follow-up period will give an imprecise estimate of the effect, which may lead to detection bias.

Recall bias

If the subject knows which treatment he has been allocated to, his decision might be influenced by his beliefs about the effectiveness of the treatment. For example, subjects who knowingly receive a new treatment for chronic pain might expect it to have a positive effect on their pain levels. These subjects are therefore more likely to perceive having less pain compared with if they were knowingly allocated to the usual treatment. This type of bias, known as participant expectation bias (a type of recall bias), can be prevented if the subjects are kept blind to their treatment allocation.

Interviewer bias

Please refer to Chapter 12 on cohort studies for a discussion on interviewer bias, which may be an issue when questioning subjects about their disease status.

INTERPRETING THE RESULTS

After randomization, individuals are followed up to ascertain whether there is an association between the intervention and outcome. As RCTs are prospective, it is possible to estimate a number of outcome measures, including:

- Risk ratio or odds ratio: The ratio of the event rate in the intervention group and in the control group (risk ratio discussed in Chapter 12 and odds ratio in Chapter 13).

Chlamydia in a sample population of 200 medical students. Subjects are examined once a year for up to 5 years. The graph shown in Fig. 14.2 illustrates the number of students diagnosed with their first attack of *Chlamydia* when subjects were examined on a yearly basis. The person-time is the sum of the total time contributed by all 200 subjects. The unit for person-time is person-years in this study. Therefore, the person-time contributed by all subjects is:

- At 1 year, there were 40 new cases, and we assume they all developed *Chlamydia* at 0.5 years, thus contributing $(40 \times 0.5) = 20$ person-years.
- At 2 years, there were 21 new cases and we assume they all developed *Chlamydia* at 1.5 years, thus contributing $(21 \times 1.5) = 31.5$ person-years.
- At 3 years, there were 15 new cases, and we assume they all developed *Chlamydia* at 2.5 years, thus contributing $(15 \times 2.5) = 37.5$ person-years.
- At 4 years, there were 10 new cases, and we assume they all developed *Chlamydia* at 3.5 years, thus contributing $(10 \times 3.5) = 35$ person-years.
- At 5 years, there were 8 new cases, and we assume they all developed *Chlamydia* at 4.5 years, thus contributing $(8 \times 4.5) = 36$ person-years.
- Accounting for the 106 people who never developed *Chlamydia* over the 5-year study period, they contributed $(106 \times 5) = 530$ person-years.
- The total time-years contributed by all subjects is 690 person-years $(= 20 + 31.5 + 37.5 + 35 + 36 + 530)$.

The incidence rate of *Chlamydia* in medical students is:

$$\frac{94}{690 \text{ person-years}} = 0.136 \text{ cases per person-year}$$

By multiplying the numerator and denominator by 1000, the incidence rate becomes 136 cases per 1000 person-years.

In other words, if you were to follow 1000 medical students for one year, you would see 136 new cases of *Chlamydia*!

Prevalence versus incidence

We can use the concept of tap water running into a sink to demonstrate the relationship between incidence and prevalence (Fig. 14.3). Prevalence can be considered as the proportion of a sink (total population) filled with water (prevalent cases). Flow of the tap water into the sink represents incident cases. Drainage of water down the sink drainpipe represents prevalent cases leaving the prevalence pool due to recovery (cure), death or emigration. Using this model, we can conclude that the prevalence increases if:

- the rate of new cases arising increases (more tap water runs into the sink).
- the number of cases who recover, die or emigrate decreases (less water drains from the sink).

A successful treatment that improves survival rates (without curing the disease) will increase the prevalence of the disease. The interrelationship between prevalence and incidence can be mathematically expressed as:

$$\text{Prevalence} = \text{Incidence rate} \times \text{Average duration of the disease}$$

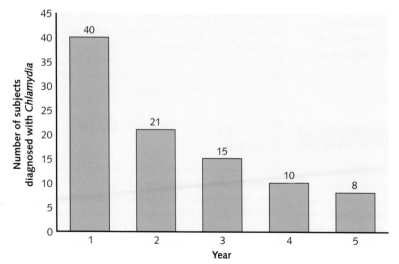

Fig. 14.2 Number of subjects diagnosed with *Chlamydia* on a yearly basis.

Fig. 14.3 Incidence versus prevalence.

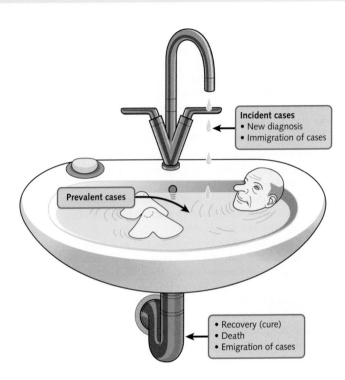

Incident cases
• New diagnosis
• Immigration of cases

Prevalent cases

• Recovery (cure)
• Death
• Emigration of cases

We assume that the prevalence of the disease in the population is low, i.e., less than 0.10, when using this formula. This formula can only be used under certain conditions, known as the steady state, which implies that:

- The length of time from diagnosis to recovery or death is stable.
- The incidence rate of the disease has been stable over time, i.e., no marked reduction of the disease or recent epidemics.

HINTS AND TIPS

The prevalence of a disease can increase, either because the disease prevalence has increased or because the average duration of the disease has increased.

STUDY DESIGN

A cross-sectional study is a form of observational study that involves collecting data from a target population at a single point in time. This methodology is particularly useful for assessing the true burden of a disease or the health needs of a population. Cross-sectional studies are therefore useful for planning the provision and allocation of health resources. Most government surveys conducted by the National Centre

for Health Statistics are cross-sectional studies. Compared with information from routine hospital or primary care health records, the data collected from cross-sectional studies are systematically collected and less subject to measurement bias. Data collection methods include questionnaires, medical examinations and interviews. While questionnaires are cheaper than interviews, the response rate is usually lower; thus a large study sample size is required when using questionnaires.

Cross-sectional studies are good at discovering people with a disease who have not previously sought any medical advice. Healthcare professionals are usually only aware of the relatively small proportion of individuals that present to them with an illness. There is often more disease in the community, irrespective of whether individuals are symptomatic (e.g., stable angina) or asymptomatic (e.g., asymptomatic HIV infection). This phenomenon is known as the clinical iceberg (Fig. 14.4). Cross-sectional studies are able to uncover the iceberg of disease.

Descriptive cross-sectional studies

Descriptive cross-sectional studies are used to measure the prevalence and distribution of a disease in a defined population. Prevalence can be assessed at a single point in time (point prevalence). For example, a random sample of medical schools across London was selected to measure the prevalence or burden of depression amongst medical students. Prevalence can also be assessed over a defined period of

Effect modification by group

Effect modification may be an issue when the rate difference for the exposure effect (at the individual level) varies across groups. Effect modification is different from confounding as instead of competing with the exposure as an aetiological factor for the disease, the effect modifier identifies subpopulations (or subgroups) that are particularly susceptible to the exposure of interest. Effect modifiers are therefore not in the causal pathway of the disease process. Ecological fallacy may be an issue if these covariate levels exist within groups.

To demonstrate this concept, let us look at the effect of smoking on the risk of developing lung cancer. It is well known that smoking and asbestos exposure are both risk factors for lung cancer. People who smoke cigarettes have a risk of developing lung cancer that is 20–25 times greater than that in nonsmokers. Nonsmokers exposed to asbestos have a three- to five-fold increased risk of developing lung cancer than those not exposed to asbestos. However, people who chronically inhaled asbestos fibres (e.g., shipyard workers) and also smoked cigarettes had about a 64-fold increased risk of developing lung cancer. Therefore, the effects of smoking and asbestos exposure are not additive, but multiplicative. There seems to be an interaction whereby the effects of smoking on the risk of developing lung cancer are magnified in people who have also been exposed to asbestos. In this example, asbestos exposure is the effect modifier.

> **HINTS AND TIPS**
>
> Unlike confounding, effect modification is a biological phenomenon whereby the effect modifier identifies subpopulations that are particularly susceptible to the exposure of interest.

Confounders and modifiers

Confounding and effect modification can arise in three distinct ways:

- The ecological exposure variable has an effect on risk that is distinct from the effect of its individual-level analogue, e.g., living in a country with national health guidelines favouring MMR vaccination versus actually having the MMR vaccine (in the autism example discussed above).
- The confounders and effect modifiers may have different patterns of distribution across the groups.
- The risk of the disease outcome may depend on the prevalence of that disease in the rest of the population in the group. This usually holds true for many infectious diseases.

These scenarios cannot be observed in ecological data and the degree of association between the exposure and outcome gives no indication of the presence, direction or magnitude of ecological bias. In an attempt to reduce the risk of ecological fallacy, some researchers use smaller geographical catchment areas (e.g., cities instead of countries) in order to make the groups more homogeneous in terms of exposure level. However, this strategy has its disadvantages:

- There is a greater chance of migration of individuals between groups. This can lead to migration bias as migrants and nonmigrants may differ on both exposure prevalence and disease risk. Studies have shown that migration can also contribute to ecological fallacy.
- Sufficient data may not be available.

> **HINTS AND TIPS**
>
> Ecological associations can differ from the corresponding associations at the individual level within groups of the same population. This underpins the reason behind ecological fallacy.

Causality

In ecological studies, the temporal relationship between the exposure and the outcome is not clear-cut as the exposure status is measured at the same time as the outcome. For a more in-depth discussion on causality, please refer to the Bradford-Hill criteria, which are discussed in Chapter 10.

Individual-level studies versus group-level studies

It is important to understand that group-level study designs sometimes surpass individual-level study designs for one of the following reasons.

Design limitations of individual-level studies

If a particular exposure varies little within a study area, individual-level studies may not be suitable for estimating the exposure effects. On the other hand, ecological studies may be able to measure significant variations in mean exposure across different geographical areas.

Measurement limitations of individual-level studies

With limited time and resource availability, we often cannot accurately measure relevant exposures at the individual level for large numbers of subjects. This usually holds true when investigating apparent clusters of disease in

Advantages of ecological studies

- Can investigate whether differences in exposure between areas are bigger than at the individual level.
- Use routinely collected health data, therefore may be relatively cheap and quick to conduct.
- Generate hypotheses that can be investigated at the individual level using studies higher up in the hierarchy of evidence.
- Can investigate the effect of exposures that are measured over groups or areas, e.g., diet, air pollution and temperature.
- Can search for associations in large populations.

Disadvantages of ecological studies

- Associations cannot be confirmed at the individual level.
- There is potential for ecological fallacy when applying grouped results to the individual level.
- There is lack of available data on confounding factors.
- There is potential for systematic differences between areas in how disease frequency is measured, e.g., differences in disease classification and coding.
- There is potential for systematic differences between areas in how exposures are measured.

small areas. On some occasions, individual-level exposures cannot be measured accurately due to considerable person-to-person variability, e.g., when measuring dietary factors. In such situations, ecological measures might accurately reflect group averages.

KEY EXAMPLE OF AN ECOLOGICAL STUDY

There is increasing evidence to suggest that determinants such as an individual's educational background or socioeconomic status may have a profound effect on their health status. However, gathering data on socioeconomic status at an individual level has proven to be very difficult as:

- it is a sensitive issue to discuss with members of the public.

- the socioeconomic status varies dramatically depending on the life course of the subject. For example, if someone has recently retired, they may have a low annual income, yet have a relatively high socioeconomic status based on income acquired during their working life.

Due to these challenges faced, ecological studies have been used to investigate the effect of socioeconomic status on various health outcomes. In these studies, we assume that the region where people live is a reflection of their socioeconomic status. These regions are usually defined using postcodes, which are linked to census information on the median household income within a given area. This approach makes the assumption that all individuals living within a defined geographical area have a similar socioeconomic status.

Relationship between socioeconomic status and mortality after an acute myocardial infarction

Alter and colleagues conducted a well-known ecological study investigating the relationship between a patient's socioeconomic status (along with access to cardiac procedures such as angioplasty and cardiac bypass grafting surgery) and mortality after an acute myocardial infarction in Ontario, Canada. Patients were categorized into five income quintiles from the lowest to the highest using the strategy described above. The research group found that patients living in higher-income neighbourhoods had the highest rates of cardiac procedure use and the lowest one-year mortality. However, this finding alone does not provide us with evidence that the socioeconomic status, the degree of access that an individual has to a cardiac procedure and the mortality after an acute myocardial infarction are causally related.

A follow-up study was therefore conducted at the individual level using clinical and socioeconomic status data. The research group showed that much of the acute myocardial infarction mortality gradient was associated with differences in the patient's baseline cardiovascular risk factor profile (and not associated with discrepancies in the degree of access that the patients had to a cardiac procedure). Consequently, we can conclude that universal healthcare for all individuals, regardless of socioeconomic status, cannot eliminate health disparities on its own. Instead, policy-makers should focus on improving the resources available to healthcare professionals to reduce the cardiovascular risk factor profile of their patients, especially among those who have a lower socioeconomic status.

HINTS AND TIPS

An association between a particular exposure and outcome (observed in an ecological study) can stimulate the need for an individual-level study in order to determine the mechanisms involved for this association.

● Chapter Summary

- An ecological study is an observational study in which the units of observation and analysis are at a group level, rather than at an individual level.
- Ecological studies are near the bottom of the hierarchy of what counts as reliable evidence for clinical decision-making.
- Using aggregate data, ecological studies examine the association between exposures and outcomes.
- The goal of an ecological study may be to make biologic inferences about effects on individual risks or to make ecological inferences about effects on group rates.
- The grouping used in ecological studies may be by time (time trend studies), place (geographical studies) or both (mixed design).
- The data collected on the exposure and outcome variables should be at the same level of aggregation (e.g., time period, city, region, country, continent).
- The results of a geographical study are usually analysed initially by looking at the strength of the association between the exposure and outcome variables.
- The Pearson correlation coefficient (r) measures the degree of linear association between two continuous variables, i.e., the exposure and outcome variables.
- The closer the value of r is to 1, the stronger the relationship between the two continuous variables.
- Ecological fallacy is a limitation commonly faced when using ecological studies to make causal inferences between an exposure and outcome and is a type of bias. Ecological fallacy occurs when correlations based on grouped data are incorrectly assumed to hold at the individual level.
- Ecological bias can result from three main sources (within-group bias, confounding by group or effect modification by group).
- The advantages and disadvantages of ecological studies covered in this chapter should be considered when writing or critiquing this type of study design.

REFERENCES

Alter, D.A., Naylor, C.D., Austin, P., Tu, J.V., 1999. Effects of socioeconomic status on access to invasive cardiac procedures and on mortality after acute myocardial infarction. N. Engl. J. Med. 341, 1359–1367.

Alter, D.A., Chong, A., Austin, P.C., Mustard, C., Iron, K., Williams, J.I., Morgan, C.D., Tu, J.V., Irvine, J., Naylor, C.D., 2006. SESAMI Study Group. Socioeconomic status and mortality after acute myocardial infarction. Ann. Intern. Med. 144 (2), 82–93.

FURTHER READING

Levin, K.A., 2006. Study Design VI – Ecological Studies. Evid. Based Dent. 7, 108.

Morgenstern, H., 2013. Ecologic studies. In: Rothman, K.J., Greenland, S., Lash, T.L. (Eds.), Modern Epidemiology, third ed. Lippincott-Raven, Philadelphia, pp. 511–531.

Morgenstern, H., 1995. Ecologic studies in epidemiology: Concepts, principles, and methods. Annu. Rev. Public Health 16, 61–81.

Case report and case series 16

BACKGROUND

According to the National Health Services Centre for Reviews and Dissemination, case reports and case series are near the bottom of the hierarchy (Chapter 2: Fig. 2.2) of what counts as reliable evidence for clinical decision-making. A case report (or case study) usually describes a single unique case or finding of interest. A case series (or clinical series):

- is a descriptive study that reports on data from a group of individuals who have a similar disease or condition.
- is a type of observational study useful for identifying similar or differing characteristics between selected cases.
- can be prospective or retrospective and usually involves only a small number of individuals.
- can include either nonconsecutive (a selection of cases) or consecutive individuals (all cases) with the same condition or disease.

The information gained from a case series can be used to generate hypotheses. Case series studies are commonly used to report on a consecutive series of patients with a defined disease who have been treated in a similar manner (without a control group).

WHAT IS THE ROLE OF CASE REPORTS AND CASE SERIES?

Most case reports and case series cover one of six topics:

1. Identifying and describing new diseases.
2. Identifying rare or unique manifestations of known diseases.
3. Audit, quality improvement and medical education.
4. Understanding the pathogenesis of a disease.
5. Detecting new drug side-effects, both beneficial and adverse.
6. Reporting unique therapeutic approaches.

CONDUCTING A CASE REPORT

Preparation

- Identify an interesting case in a clinic or on the ward, with guidance and advice from a senior colleague.
- Having identified a suitable case, carry out a literature review to explore the uniqueness of the case. Have similar cases already been published?

- Discuss the case with senior doctors who have been looking after the patient in order to gain permission and support.
- Gain written consent from the patient, especially if there may be patient identifiers in the report, including medical pictures and specific clinical details.
- Some journals require patient consent regardless of whether or not patient identifiers are included in the report, so read the journal guidelines carefully!
- Having successfully completed the above, relevant information should be gathered about the case from the patient notes, available imaging, laboratory results and other relevant sources.

Structuring a medical case report

The following guideline for writing a case report manuscript can also be used as a checklist when critically appraising case studies already published.

Abstract

There is usually a strict word limit for the abstract, so carefully read the journal guidelines before you begin! The abstract will help readers discern whether they are interested (or not interested) in reading the case report. The abstract should include all the sections included in the main text of the case report, including the introduction and objective(s), case presentation, discussion and conclusion. The abstract should be engaging and to the point, highlighting the key details from the main text of the case report.

Introduction

The opening sentence should be catchy and attract the attention of the reader. The subject matter of interest should be introduced with background information on the topic. The search strategy for the literature review, including the search terms used, should be described with enough detail to allow the reader to reproduce the search easily. The purpose and merit of the case report should be highlighted using the literature identified in the search. The patient case should be introduced to the reader with a one- or two-sentence description. There should not be more than three or four concise paragraphs for the introduction of the case report.

Case presentation

The case should be described in enough detail to allow readers to make their own conclusions about the case. Patient identifiers such as precise dates and the patient's date of birth should be avoided. A narrative description of the case should be written with significant events discussed in chronological order (headings for each part of the patient history should not be used). The patient information described should be relevant and may include details on:

- Patient demographics: age, sex, race, height and weight.
- Presenting complaint.
- Past medical history.
- Drug history before and during admission (include over-the-counter medications, recreational drugs, vaccines and herbal remedies): the name, dose, route, times of administration and compliance rates of all medications should be listed.
- Renal and hepatic function: allows assessment of the appropriateness of the medication doses used.
- Drug allergies: including the name of culprit medications, the date and type of drug reactions.
- Family history.
- Social history: diet, occupation, smoking and alcohol status.
- Important physical examination findings.
- Relevant (not routine) laboratory data.
- Differential diagnoses and the diagnostic procedure.
- Report the results of any diagnostic tests.
- Therapeutic effects and side-effects of any treatments on the disease outcome.
- Potential causal relationships between an exposure and outcome.
- Current status of the patient case and future treatment plans.

Relevant figures should be used, including electrocardiograms, radiological images, blood films and photographs of skin manifestations.

Discussion

- What new information has been learnt from the case report?
- Comment on how unique the case is by comparing and contrasting it to other cases already published in the literature.
- Are there any inaccuracies in the data that would question the validity of the case report?
- What are the limitations of the case report?
- The key points raised from the case report should be summarized.

Conclusion

- A justified, sound and brief conclusion should be written based on information reviewed as part of the discussion.
- Any recommendations should be based on evidence rather than speculation.
- A description should be provided on whether any new findings from the case will have an impact on clinical practice.
- Has the case report generated any novel hypotheses that could be investigated using a study higher up in the hierarchy of evidence?

References

Whether other articles are quoted or paraphrased, it is essential that all sources of information referred to in the case report be acknowledged in the reference section at the end of the paper. Please refer to Chapter 10 for an in depth discussion on the common referencing systems used. Citations should be included in parentheses in the main text of the case report.

CONDUCTING A CASE SERIES

Guidelines similar to those outlined for case reports should be followed when conducting a case series. However, specifically for case series, it is important to consider the following:

- Is the case series prospective or retrospective? Prospective case series are less prone to bias.
- Case series should be carried out according to a predefined protocol, which clearly defines all stages of the study, including patient selection, measures, data collection, analysis and reporting.
- Inclusion and exclusion criteria should be clearly defined, with all eligible patients selected in order to avoid selection bias.
- Are nonconsecutive or consecutive cases selected? Recruiting consecutive cases is preferable in order to avoid selection bias.
- Are patients recruited over a fixed time period or (preferably) until a sufficient number of cases are identified? Formal sample size calculations could be used if a particular change in measure is worth demonstrating.
- The diagnostic process should be clearly documented for all patients.
- Details of baseline information and pretreatment and posttreatment measures should be recorded.
- The outcome for all study participants should be measured in the same way according to the predefined protocol.
- Outcomes should be measured objectively, wherever possible, in order to minimize measurement bias.
- Measurements made should be valid and reliable.
- Differences in treatment effects should be compared and contrasted between cases.
- Quantitative data should be statistically analysed, for example, by calculating the average value (the mean) and the degree of spread of the data set (e.g., the standard deviation or interquartile range).
- The 'flow of patients' should be described, accounting for anyone who dropped out of the study, therefore avoiding selection bias (please refer to Chapter 12 for a discussion on selection bias).
- An intention-to-treat analysis should be considered where appropriate (please refer to Chapter 11 for a discussion on how to calculate and interpret the intention-to-treat analysis).

Quota sampling

Quota sampling is sometimes considered a type of purposive sampling. The decision on how many people with certain characteristics to include as study participants is made during the design phase of the study. These characteristics include gender, age, socioeconomic class, marital status, profession, disease status, etc. The characteristics chosen are to identify people most likely to have insight or have experienced the research topic. Individuals from the community are then recruited until the predefined quota is satisfied.

COMMON PITFALLS

THE DIFFERENCE BETWEEN PURPOSIVE AND QUOTA SAMPLING

While the aim of both purposive and quota sampling is to identify study participants who satisfy predefined criteria, quota sampling is more specific with regards to sample size. For example, you may be interested in investigating gender-specific responses to a new diagnosis of colon cancer. Assuming there is a 1:1 gender ratio in the population, the aim of a quota sample would be to identify an equal number of men and women with colon cancer in the population. On the other hand, purposive sampling would involve setting a target for the number of participants in each group, rather than a strict quota.

Snowball sampling

Snowball sampling (also known as chain referral sampling) involves using study participants as informants to identify other people who could potentially participate in the study. The study participants, with whom contact has already been made, use their social networks to identify groups not easily accessible to researchers, such as the homeless.

Maximum variation sampling

Maximum variation sampling involves selecting people to obtain a broad range of perspectives on the research topic. In other words, the aim of maximum variation sampling is to increase the diversity of the perspectives obtained. For example, you may be interested in investigating patient responses to a new diagnosis of cancer. Maximum variation sampling would involve recruiting patients with different demographic profiles, e.g., age, ethnicity, gender, as well as including patients who have different types of cancer.

Negative sampling

Negative sampling (also known as deviant case sampling) involves searching for unusual or atypical cases of the research topic of interest. For example, you may be interested in interviewing women who had a positive cervical screen for cervical intraepithelial neoplasia. Negative sampling would also involve interviewing those women who tested negative to see whether their views about the cervical screening process differ.

ORGANIZING AND ANALYSING THE DATA

Organizing the data

Organizing data in a standardized way is essential to ensure the validity of the study results. Despite being a challenging process, qualitative data needs to be systematically compared and analysed in its raw form. Soon after collecting the data:

- the field notes should be expanded into a descriptive narrative of what was observed. The narrative is usually typed into computer files.
- audio recordings should be transcribed.

Any initial observations should be elaborated in as much detail as possible, describing what happened and what was learnt from:

- the setting and study population (during participant observation).
- the interview content, the participant(s) and the context (during one-to-one interviews and focus groups).

Narrative accounts and typed transcripts are subsequently coded according to the particular responses to each question and/or to common emerging themes.

Analysing the data

Following the research question as a guide, every line of text is coded for relevant themes. Coding is the process of collecting observations into groups that are like one another and assigning a symbol, known as a code, as a name for the group. As themes/categories are developed, the researcher assigns a working definition to each code. This definition is continually being challenged when going through the text. Using this process, new codes are developed when the properties of the current codes do not fit the text. Furthermore, codes that are rarely used are dismissed.

As highlighted previously, there is usually a constant cycle of collecting data, analysing the data, generating codes and themes/categories and then collecting more data to refine our understanding of the topic until saturation is achieved. This constant comparison approach is therefore iterative (moving back and forth) and inductive (a type of reasoning that involves extrapolating patterns from the data in order to form a conceptual category/theme). The analysis is grounded in the categories or theories generated from the data. Software data management packages are available to assist with the analysis. The ultimate goal of the analysis is to generate analytical concepts that can be used to generate new hypotheses.

VALIDITY, RELIABILITY AND TRANSFERABILITY

There are three key concepts that need to be considered when appraising a qualitative research paper:

1. Validity: The degree to which the findings accurately represent the specific concept that the researcher is attempting to measure.
2. Reliability: Would another researcher be able to reproduce the same data and interpret them in the same way?
3. Transferability: Are the findings applicable to other patients and/or settings?

Validity

The setting and method used for data collection should be justified. For example, if investigating how patients with breast cancer want their doctors to communicate with them, study participants should be interviewed, on a one-to-one basis, but not on hospital premises. Carrying out interviews away from the hospital, for example, at the patient's home, will allow study participants to feel more at ease, thus giving them an opportunity to discuss any negative feelings that they might have. All data collected should be analysed, even if negative attitudes are portrayed. The final report should include quotes that highlight both positive and negative experiences.

The researcher should reflect on whether his or her values and attributes may have influenced (or biased) any stages of the study. This is often referred to as 'reflexivity'. For example, an 18-year-old man and a 50-year-old woman are likely to elicit different responses to questions about sexual health when interviewing a group of teenagers. The values and attributes considered may include:

- ethnicity
- gender
- age
- whether the researcher has the same condition as the one being investigated.

The findings from the study (i.e., analytical categories/themes) should be well grounded in the data. Did the researchers use the constant comparison method to clarify the emerging themes? Sufficient raw data should be included in the final report to enable the reader to draw the same conclusions as the researchers. The report should therefore include direct quotes from the study participants. Some studies show evidence of triangulation, which involves cross-verifying the research findings by using more than one research method. The major types of triangulation involve:

- having multiple researchers in the study
- using more than one method to gather data
- recruiting a range of patients from different backgrounds.

A research finding is accepted more readily if various methods lead to the same finding.

Reliability

Similar to our discussion for validity, the setting and method used for data collection should be justified. If the issue of reflexivity has not been considered, another researcher might obtain different findings if the research study was repeated. The codes and themes should be derived from the data, i.e., using the actual words of the participants. If they were derived from the researcher's own beliefs, other researchers might obtain different codes and themes if they tried to replicate the research study. In an attempt to ensure that the codes and themes are derived from the data, some research groups get a second researcher to code the data independently, thus checking for inter-rater reliability.

Transferability

After ensuring that the study findings are valid and reliable, the final step is to consider whether they can be applied to other patients and settings. Assessing transferability does not involve carrying out statistical calculations, as is the case for quantitative research. Instead, you must assess whether the nature of the sample and the study setting have been described in enough detail to allow readers to determine whether the findings can be applied to their patients and settings.

ADVANTAGES AND DISADVANTAGES

What are the advantages and disadvantages of qualitative research?

Advantages of qualitative research

- Can use a personal approach to investigate sensitive issues, e.g., mental health and sexual health.
- Can investigate the views of people usually excluded from surveys, e.g., individuals with dementia or learning difficulties.
- Can investigate processes by exploring answers to how and why questions.
- Can discover issues that are important from the perspective of those being studied, e.g., patients and healthcare professionals.
- Can investigate behaviours, opinions, beliefs, experiences and emotions of individuals.
- Can investigate how an individual's social environment influences behaviour.

Disadvantages of qualitative research

- Researcher bias is inherent in this type of study design and is sometimes unavoidable.
- Compared with quantitative studies, it is more difficult to determine the validity and reliability of qualitative research data.
- The study sample may not be representative of the larger population.
- It takes time for the researcher to build trust with the study participants in order to facilitate full self-representation.
- Data collection using participant observation is time-consuming and potentially expensive and requires a well-trained researcher.
- Transcribing recorded findings is time-consuming and labour intensive.
- Using an in-depth, comprehensive approach to gathering data limits the scope of the findings.

KEY EXAMPLE OF QUALITATIVE RESEARCH

Research has shown that doctors often communicate poorly with patients who have cancer. Systematic research into patients' perspectives can guide future development of communication training for clinicians specializing in cancer. In 2004, Emma Wright and her colleagues carried out a qualitative study to determine how patients with breast cancer want their doctors to communicate with them. Thirty-nine women with primary breast cancer were selected from surgery and oncology clinics.

Clinical consultations were recorded and semistructured interviews carried out in the patient's own home, thus making the participants feel more at ease. In an attempt to minimize idealized or generalized accounts, the semistructured interviews were carried out within 1–5 days of the patient's consultation. Considering there are two sources for data collection (recorded consultations and semistructured interviews), there is evidence of triangulation. Importantly, the interviewer explained that she was a researcher, independent of the clinical team. The transcript from the patient's clinical consultation was shown to the patient during the interview to help her describe those aspects of the doctor–patient communication that she valued or deprecated. The interviewer used open-ended questions, prompts and reflection during the interview.

Anonymized interview transcripts were analysed inductively, in parallel with the interviews, using a constant comparison approach. By using data collection and data analysis, recurrent patterns were identified. The transcripts were reviewed by two researchers, thus taking into account inter-rater reliability. The study ended when the saturation point was achieved. Using the constant-comparison approach, the codes and categories derived from the data were well grounded. Some of the codes identified for the category 'Ways in which doctors could communicate expertise' include:

- Demonstrate a tangible skill.
- Display confidence and efficiency and make things happen.
- Answer all questions without hesitation.
- Do not mislead.
- Tell the patient you will be open.

Furthermore, the paper presented sufficient raw data to enable the reader to generate similar codes. Overall, as highlighted, this study addresses issues regarding the validity and reliability of the findings. Are the findings applicable to other patients/settings? To address issues regarding the transferability of the findings, the research group presented a table that summarized the characteristics of the patients and doctors whose consultations were recorded.

> ● **Chapter Summary**
>
> - Qualitative research seeks to understand the research question or topic from the perspectives of the local population involved.
> - Qualitative research allows us to obtain information on the actions, behaviours, values and opinions of different groups in the population, e.g., from different cultures, socioeconomic classes or genders.
> - The three most commonly used qualitative research methods are participant observation, in-depth interviews and focus groups.
> - Participant observation is suitable when collecting data on naturally occurring behaviours of participants in their usual setting.
> - In-depth interviews are suitable when collecting data on the participants' perspectives and experiences in relation to the research topic.
> - Focus groups are suitable when collecting data on the cultural norms of various groups.
> - Qualitative research is usually based on selecting small samples (i.e., a subset of the population) to investigate a particular topic in depth and detail.
> - While the aim of both purposive and quota sampling is to identify study participants who satisfy predefined criteria, quota sampling is more specific with regards to sample size.
> - Snowball sampling involves using study participants as informants to identify other people who could potentially participate in the study.
> - Maximum variation sampling involves selecting people to obtain a broad range of perspectives on the research topic.
> - Negative sampling involves searching for unusual or atypical cases of the research topic of interest.
> - Narrative accounts and typed transcripts are coded according to the particular responses to each question and/or to common emerging themes.
> - When appraising a qualitative research paper, it is important to consider the validity, reliability and transferability of the study.
> - Validity refers to the degree to which the findings accurately represent the specific concept that the researcher is attempting to measure.
> - Reliability answers the question of whether another researcher would be able to reproduce the same data and interpret them in a similar way.
> - Transferability answers the question of whether the study findings are applicable to other patients and/or settings.
> - The advantages and disadvantages of qualitative research covered in this chapter should also be considered when writing or critiquing this type of study design.

REFERENCES

Wright, E.B., Holcombe, C., Salmon, P., 2004. Doctors' communication of trust, care and respect in breast cancer: qualitative study. BMJ 328 (7444), 864.

Glaser, B.G., Strauss, A.L., 1967. Discovery of Grounded Theory: Strategies for Qualitative Research. Aldine, Chicago.

Mack, N., Woodsong, C., MacQueen, K.M., Guest, G., Namey, E., 2005. Qualitative Research Methods: A Data Collector's Field Guide. Family Health International, North Carolina.

Sutton, J., Austin, Z., 2015. Qualitative research: data collection, analysis, and management. Can. J. Hosp. Pharm. 68 (3), 226–231.

FURTHER READING

Barbour, R., 2001. Checklists for improving rigour in qualitative research: A case of the tail wagging the dog? BMJ 322, 1115–1117.

Britten, N., 1995. Qualitative research: qualitative interviews in medical research. BMJ 311, 251–253.

Confounding | 18

WHAT IS CONFOUNDING?

Confounding:

- occurs when the association between an exposure and disease outcome is distorted by a third variable, which is known as a confounder (Fig. 18.1);
- is a form of bias as it can lead to an over- or underestimation of the observed association between an exposure and disease outcome;
- may be an issue in both observational and experimental studies (randomized controlled trials);
- is more likely to occur in observational studies than in randomised controlled trials.

As subjects are randomly allocated to exposed and unexposed groups in experimental studies, both groups are expected to be comparable with regard to known and unknown confounding factors. However, there may be random differences between the exposed and unexposed groups, which may potentially lead to confounding. In observational studies, in addition to random differences between the exposed and unexposed groups, variables related to the exposure may confound the association between the exposure and disease outcome. Of all study designs, ecological studies are the most susceptible to confounding due to the difficulty in controlling for confounders at a group level. Provided the confounding factors are recognized and

measured at the start of the study, they may be controlled for at the study design level or when analysing the results of the study.

ASSESSING FOR POTENTIAL CONFOUNDING FACTORS

Potential confounders should be working independently of the exposure–disease association pathway. To decide whether this is the case, there must be a social or biological mechanism to link the exposure to the disease outcome. These mechanisms are based on the available evidence from previous clinical or nonclinical findings.

Association with exposure

The confounding factor will be associated with the exposure with at least one of the following relationships.

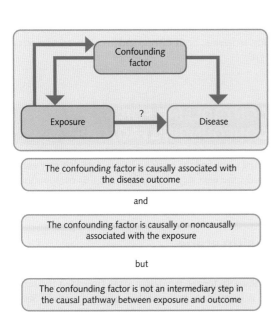

Fig. 18.1 Schematic of confounding.

The confounder causes the exposure

- *Research question:* Is hypertension associated with mortality rates independent of levels of exercise?
- *Biological mechanism linking exposure to outcome:* Hypertension increases mortality rate due to an increased risk of ischaemic heart disease.
- *Potential confounder:* Physical inactivity.

A person's level of physical activity may be a confounder in the relationship between hypertension and mortality, because physical inactivity is associated with both the exposure (hypertension) and the disease outcome (high mortality). Therefore, in this particular example, the confounder causes both the exposure and the outcome (Fig. 18.2A).

The confounder is a result of the exposure

- *Research question:* Is low social class associated with ischaemic heart disease independent of smoking status?
- *Social mechanism linking exposure to outcome:* Lower social class groups have an increased risk of ischaemic heart disease due to poor access to healthcare.
- *Potential confounder:* Smoking.

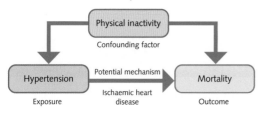

A The confounder causes the exposure

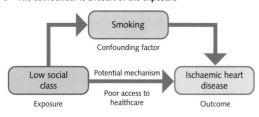

B The confounder is a result of the exposure

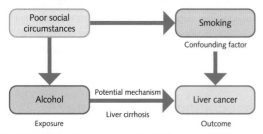

C The confounder is related to the exposure with a non-causal association (but neither causes the other)

Fig. 18.2 Schematic of association between confounding and the exposure.

168

A person's smoking status may be a confounder in the relationship between being a member of a low social class and ischaemic heart disease, because smoking is associated with both the exposure (low social class) and the disease outcome (ischaemic heart disease). Therefore, in this particular example, the exposure causes the confounder while the confounder causes the outcome (Fig. 18.2B).

The confounder is related to the exposure with a noncausal association (but neither causes the other)

- *Research question:* Is alcohol associated with liver cancer independent of smoking?
- *Biological mechanism linking exposure to outcome:* Excess alcohol is associated with primary liver cancer, through causing liver cirrhosis.
- *Potential confounder:* Smoking.

A person's smoking status may be a confounder in the relationship between alcohol and liver cancer, via a noncausal relationship. In this example, poor social circumstances, such as poverty, may cause someone to both drink alcohol and smoke. Smoking has also been shown to be a risk factor for liver cancer. Therefore, in this particular example, the confounder and the exposure are related via a noncausal separate pathway. As with all confounding factors, the confounder also causes the outcome (Fig. 18.2C).

Association with disease

In order to cause confounding, a factor must be causally associated with the disease outcome in both exposed and unexposed individuals. In all of the examples illustrated in Fig. 18.2, the confounding variables (physical inactivity and smoking) determine the likelihood of the outcome (mortality, ischaemic heart disease and liver cancer) to a certain degree.

CONTROLLING FOR CONFOUNDING FACTORS

Having identified the confounding factors that may exist in a study, the next step is to control for this confounding at either the study design level or when analysing the results of the study.

Design stage

It is sometimes important to control for very strong confounding factors at the design stage (provided the sample size is large) than at the analysis stage of a study. Several different methods may be used to minimize the degree of confounding in a study, including:

- randomization
- restriction
- matching

These methods are not exclusive to each other; therefore, more than one of these methods may be used in the same study.

Randomization

As mentioned above, randomly allocating subjects to the exposed and unexposed groups will control for both known and unknown confounders. For example, if individuals are randomly classified into two groups, the rules of probability state that both groups will have a similar distribution of confounders (especially when large sample sizes are used). Each study participant will have an equal chance of being allocated to either group. Therefore, in theory, each group will have an equal percentage of males, an equal percentage of overweight people, an equal number of women with red nail polish and so forth. The only difference between the two groups is therefore the exposure status. However, even if the sample size is large and the randomization process is unbiased, there may be random differences between the exposed and unexposed groups, which may potentially lead to confounding.

HINTS AND TIPS

The randomization process involves allocating study participants to either the exposed or unexposed group. However, in observational studies (e.g., cohort, case–control, cross-sectional and ecological), we observe subjects' exposure patterns without attempting to change them, so we cannot use randomization to control for confounding in these study designs.

Restriction

Restricting study participants to those people from the population who have not been exposed to one or more confounding factors will control for confounding caused by these variables. For example, in a study investigating whether alcohol use is associated with liver cancer independent of smoking (illustrated in Fig. 18.2C), the investigators could restrict the study population to nonsmokers. When there are strong confounding factors distorting the association between an exposure and disease outcome, restriction is ideal as it can be a useful, inexpensive and efficient method of controlling for the confounder of interest. However, there are instances when restriction is logistically

unfeasible as, following exclusion of subjects with the confounding factor, the remaining study population from which cases are selected may be too small, thus reducing the power of the study. Unfortunately, the findings from a study using this method of control for confounding cannot be generalized to those who were left out by the restriction process, thus reducing the applicability of the findings.

Matching

Matching on the confounding variable(s) is a statistical technique commonly used in observational studies, especially in case–control studies. Matching constrains subjects in both the exposed and unexposed groups to have the same value of potential confounders, such as sex and age. For example, in a study published in 2012, Driver and colleagues carried out a case–control study evaluating the relation between dementia and subsequent cancer. They matched each dementia case with up to three controls of the same sex and age who were free of dementia at the time of dementia diagnosis of the case. The cost of a study is usually lowered with matching, as a smaller sample size will be needed to carry out the study with the same degree of power. The feasibility and precision of carrying out a study can generally be increased with matching on the confounding variable(s). However, matching has certain disadvantages:

- The more variables that are matched for, the more demanding it will be to identify a sufficient number of matched subjects.
- The effect of the matching variables on the disease outcome cannot be investigated during the statistical analysis.
- If there are missing data for the case or control in a matched pair, the data from both subjects are excluded from the statistical analysis.

Analysis stage

Once the study data have been collected, there are two options for controlling for confounding factors at the analysis stage:

1. Stratified analysis
2. Mathematical modelling.

Stratified analysis

We can estimate the association between the exposure and disease outcome separately for different levels (strata) of the confounding variable (e.g., in the example illustrated in Fig. 18.2B, we would create two subgroups, smokers and nonsmokers). The separate estimates of the measure of association for each subgroup are combined to calculate the 'adjusted' measure of association (e.g., risk ratio adjusted for confounding). Although there are many methods for calculating the 'adjusted' measure of association using stratified analysis, the Mantel–Haenszel method is the most commonly used pooling procedure. Stratified analysis is usually employed to control for confounding when there are only a few confounders, i.e., three confounders. However, stratified analysis may be problematic, as the subgroups created may be too small and hence the power to detect a significant effect will be low. Furthermore, false-positive results may arise if multiple hypotheses are tested in each subgroup. In other words, the type 1 error rate (please refer to Chapter 8 for a discussion on type 1 error) increases as the number of comparisons made increases.

Mathematical modelling

Mathematical modelling is useful when simultaneously adjusting for many confounding factors in a study (e.g., the odds ratio calculated in a case–control study investigating an association between drinking carbonated drinks high in aspartame and Parkinson disease may be adjusted for age, social class, smoking and sex). Simultaneous control of two or more confounding factors can give different results from those calculated by controlling for each confounding factor individually. Calculating the 'adjusted' measure of association between an exposure and disease (by assessing the confounding factors simultaneously) better models the natural environment where the exposure, disease and confounding factors all coexist, than does controlling for each confounding factor individually. Although there are various types of mathematical models, the most commonly used model used to control for multiple confounders is logistic regression.

REPORTING AND INTERPRETING THE RESULTS

When critically appraising any observational study, it is important to consider whether the investigators accounted for the effects of confounding at the design and/or analysis stage of the study. In those studies where confounding is controlled for at the analysis stage, it is usual to display the 'crude' measure of association (i.e., before potential confounding factors are taken into account) as well as the 'adjusted' measure of association (i.e., after correcting for distortions in the data caused by confounding). If the adjusted measure of association is significantly different from the crude measure of association, then confounding is present.

It is useful to report the cut-off used to select which confounding factors are adjusted for (e.g., 10%, 20% or 30% change from crude to adjusted). If the measure of association is adjusted by less than 10% after controlling for confounding, it would be unlikely that this influence would be taken into account. The more variables that are controlled for, the wider the confidence interval will be for the measure of association (please refer to Chapter 8 for a discussion on confidence intervals), and therefore the less precise the study results will be. Age and sex are two confounding factors that are usually controlled for in every study due to the association of these variables with disease and mortality rate.

KEY EXAMPLE OF STUDY CONFOUNDING

- *Study type:* Case–control study (hypothetical).
- *Research question:* Does playing first-person shooter video games (for at least 15 hours per week) improve your ability in being able to successfully manage acute medical scenarios in an exam situation?
- *Biological mechanism linking exposure to outcome:* Playing first-person shooters improves your ability in being able to successfully manage acute medical scenarios (and therefore pass the exam) as:
  - Online play over the intercom with other players to decide the plan of attack on how to ambush the enemy will improve team-working, decision-making and delegating skills.
  - Tapping the L1 button on the joystick as fast you can in order to sprint to help your team member will improve manual dexterity.
- *Potential confounder:* Hours spent revising for the exam, age and sex.

The number of hours spent revising for the exam may be a confounder in the association between the exposure and outcome via a noncausal relationship. How active your social life is will affect the number of hours you play video games and the amount of time spent revising for the exam. Furthermore, as we all know, the more hours spent revising for an exam, the more likely you are to pass the exam! A person's age and sex may also influence both the exposure and outcome (Fig. 18.3). Table 18.1 summarizes the crude and adjusted odds ratio for the association between playing video games and exam success. The following conclusions can be drawn from the data:

- The crude odds ratio of 9.12 suggests that people who played at least 15 hours of first-person shooter video games per week had an approximately nine-times greater chance/odds of passing the acute medical scenario exam.
- Before you head towards the games console, the adjusted odds ratio of 0.94 suggests that the apparent

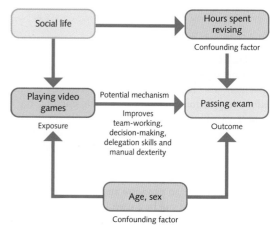

Fig. 18.3 Schematic of association.

Disadvantages of screening 👎

- A false sense of security if cases are missed (i.e., a false-negative screening result), which may delay the final diagnosis.
- Those tested negative may feel they have avoided the disease and therefore continue with their risk behaviour; for example, an individual who eats more than his recommended daily allowance of saturated fat may continue to do so if his cholesterol is within the normal range when tested by his general practitioner. Looking at the bigger picture, this may undermine primary prevention programmes; for example, to prevent coronary artery disease by promoting healthy eating.
- For cases that are true positives, treatment of early disease may be associated with potential side effects, even though the disease may not have actually progressed.
- Involves using medical resources and substantial amounts of money that could be used elsewhere, especially as the majority of people screened do not need treatment.
- Stress and anxiety caused by false alarms (i.e., a false-positive screening result). The stress may be related to unnecessary investigations, especially if it involves an invasive procedure.

Selection bias

People who participate in screening programmes often have different characteristics from those who do not. For example, when screening women aged between 50 and 70 years for breast cancer, those women with a family history of breast cancer are more likely than other women to join the mammography screening programme. Consequently, there would be higher rates of morbidity/mortality amongst this select population than in the general population. The screening test would therefore be associated with a worse prognosis and will look worse than it actually is. On the other hand, if the screening programme is more accessible to young and healthy individuals, there would be lower rates of morbidity/mortality amongst this select population than in the general population. The screening test would therefore be associated with a better prognosis and will look better than it actually is.

Length time bias

Length time bias occurs when screening tests selectively detect slowly developing cases, which have a long presymptomatic (or preclinical) phase; for example, less aggressive cancers associated with a better prognosis. The data are therefore skewed. For example, referring to Fig. 19.2, let's look at length time bias in the context of cancer screening. In general, fast-growing tumours have a shorter preclinical phase than slow-growing tumours. Therefore, there is a shorter phase during which the tumour is asymptomatic in the body (and therefore a shorter phase during which the tumour may be detected via screening). These aggressive tumours may become symptomatic in-between screening events, during which the patient may seek medical care and be diagnosed without screening. Putting this all together, if there are equal numbers of slow- and fast-growing tumours in a year, the screening test will detect more slow-growing cases (demonstrated in Fig. 19.2). Assuming that the slow-growing tumours are less likely to be fatal than the fast-growing tumours, the tumour cases detected through screening will have a better prognosis, on average, than those individuals who are diagnosed when the tumour becomes symptomatic. Screening is therefore unfairly favoured.

Lead-time bias

The intention of screening is to diagnose a disease during its preclinical phase. Without screening, the disease may only be discovered later, when the disease becomes symptomatic. Consequently, through screening, survival time (the time from diagnosis to death) appears to increase due to earlier diagnosis, even if there is no change in the disease prognosis. By analysing the raw statistics, screening will appear to increase the survival time. As shown in Fig. 19.3, this gain is called lead time. Referring to Fig. 19.3:

- Suppose the biological onset of a particular disease is at the same time in both Case 1 and Case 2.
- Case 1 is diagnosed through screening in the preclinical phase of the disease and survives for 6 years from diagnosis.
- Case 2 is diagnosed only when the subject becomes symptomatic, 4 years after Case 1 was diagnosed, and survives for 2 years from diagnosis.
- Therefore, it seems as if Case 1 survives for three-times as long as Case 2 (6 versus 2 years).
- However, the life span has not been prolonged, as both cases survive for the same amount of time since the *biological onset* of the disease.

Therefore, if early diagnosis of a disease has no effect on its biological course, lead time bias can affect the interpretation of survival rates; for example, the 5-year survival rate.

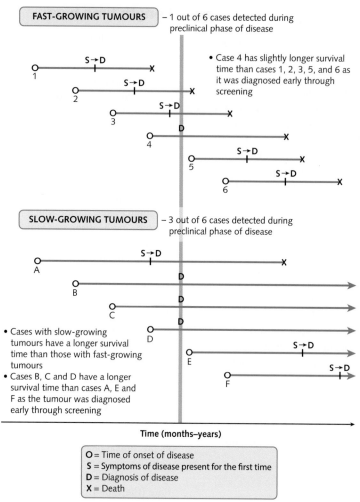

Fig. 19.2 Length time bias.

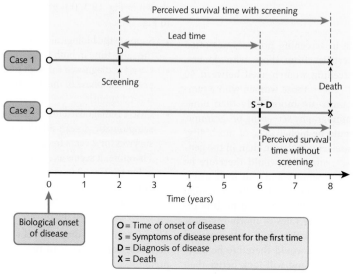

Fig. 19.3 Lead-time bias.

EXAMPLE OF A SCREENING TEST USING LIKELIHOOD RATIOS

Suppose a 60-year-old woman has a positive mammogram and asks you, her clinician, whether she has breast cancer. You explain that further testing is required; however, your patient wants to know the actual probability of her having breast cancer. Fortunately, you read this book and carry out the following calculations:

Regardless of the mammogram result, the clinician knows that the prevalence of breast cancer in the population is approximately 0.8%. A recent study has shown that the sensitivity and specificity of mammography testing in being able to detect breast cancer is 95% and 88.8%, respectively.

The pretest probability is 0.008 or 0.8%:

$$\text{Pretest odds} = \frac{\text{Pretest probability}}{1 - \text{Pretest probability}}$$

$$= \frac{0.008}{1 - 0.008}$$

$$= 0.00806$$

The likelihood ratio of breast cancer if the mammogram test is positive is:

$$\frac{\text{Sensitivity}}{1 - \text{Specificity}} = \frac{0.95}{1 - 0.888} = 8.50$$

The posttest odds in a person with a positive result are:

$$\text{Posttest odds} = \text{Pretest odds} \times \text{Positive likelihood ratio}$$
$$= 0.00806 \times 8.50 = 0.0684$$

The posttest odds can be converted back into a probability:

$$\text{Posttest probability} = \frac{\text{Posttest odds}}{\text{Posttest odds} + 1}$$

$$= \frac{0.0684}{0.0684 + 1}$$

$$= 0.064$$

$$= 6.4\%$$

An alternative approach would be to use the Fagan nomogram to work out the posttest probability (Fig. 19.4). Please refer to the text describing Fig. 19.8 for a discussion of the Fagan nomogram.

You can explain to your patient that, based on this positive mammogram, she has a 6.4% probability of having breast cancer. Therefore, a positive mammogram screening test is in itself poor at confirming breast cancer and further investigations must be undertaken.

With a sensitivity of 95%, the screening test has correctly identified 95% of all breast cancers. Furthermore, with a specificity of 88.8%, 11.2% of positive test results will be false positives (100% − 88.8%).

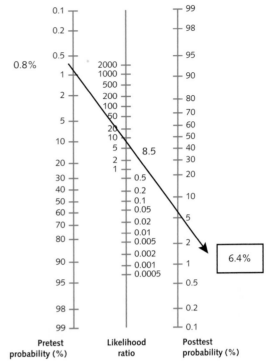

Fig. 19.4 Using the Fagan nomogram.

DIAGNOSTIC TESTS

A diagnostic test can be used to determine whether a patient is likely to have:

- a particular disease or condition (we will focus on this type of diagnostic test in this section)
- a high risk of disease; for example, checking the serum lipids in the assessment of cardiovascular disease risk
- been exposed to a particular factor; for example, paracetamol levels in an individual suspected to have taken an overdose.

Identifying new diagnostic tests may be necessary if the definitive gold standard test is expensive, invasive, risky, painful or time consuming. Diagnostic tests are not always correct 100% of the time. As clinicians rely on these diagnostic tests to make decisions on which patients need treatment, the performance (or validity) of a new test must be properly assessed before implementing its use in the clinical setting. This assessment is usually made by comparing the results of the new diagnostic test to the patient's true disease status (as assessed using the 'gold standard' test). For example, how valid is an exercise stress test (also known as an exercise EKG) for diagnosing coronary artery disease (CAD; usually >50% fixed coronary artery stenosis) compared with the gold standard test used for cardiac testing, angiography? The four key measures used to evaluate the performance of a new test are:

- sensitivity
- specificity
- positive predictive value (PPV)
- negative predictive value (NPV).

EVALUATING THE PERFORMANCE OF A DIAGNOSTIC TEST

Sensitivity and specificity

Suppose we carry out a study to evaluate the performance of a new diagnostic test for a particular disease. Each person taking this test will either have or not have the disease. However, there are four possible types of outcomes of a diagnostic test:

1. *True positive*: People with the disease who are correctly diagnosed as having the disease.
2. *False positive* (also known as 'type I error'): People without the disease who are incorrectly identified as having the disease.
3. *True negative*: People without the disease who are correctly identified as being disease free.
4. *False negative* (also known as 'type II error'): People with the disease who are incorrectly identified as being disease free.

Assuming the diagnostic test can only be positive or negative, indicating the presence or absence of disease, we can draw up a 2 × 2 table of frequencies for the different types of outcomes discussed above (Table 19.2). The sensitivity and specificity are measures that assess the validity of diagnostic tests.

Sensitivity describes the ability of the test to correctly identify people *with* the disease; i.e., the percentage of individuals with the disease who have positive test results. The sensitivity of a test can be written as:

$$\text{Sensitivity} = \frac{\text{True positive}}{\text{True positive} + \text{False negative}}$$
$$= \frac{\text{TP}}{\text{TP} + \text{FN}}$$

Specificity describes the ability of the test to correctly identify people *without* the disease; i.e., the percentage of individuals without the disease who have negative test results. The specificity of a test can be written as:

$$\text{Specificity} = \frac{\text{True negative}}{\text{True negative} + \text{False positive}}$$
$$= \frac{\text{TN}}{\text{TP} + \text{FP}}$$

An ideal test would be both highly sensitive and highly specific, where disease would be correctly identified in 100% of those individuals who truly have the disease (100% sensitivity) and disease would be ruled out in 100% of those individuals who truly don't have the disease (100% specificity). However, it is often difficult in reality to have a diagnostic test that is high in both sensitivity and specificity.

For any test, there is usually a trade-off between the sensitivity and specificity. Fig. 19.5 demonstrates this point with the use of test result distribution curves. Referring to Fig. 19.5A, the two distributions represent the results of the diagnostic test (which consist of a continuous measurement) in individuals who do and do not have the disease. The threshold of the test is the cut-off used in declaring that the test is positive. The investigator can adjust the threshold (black vertical line in Fig. 19.5B), which will in turn alter the sensitivity and specificity of the test. Increasing the threshold (by shifting) the vertical line to the right increases the specificity but decreases the sensitivity of the diagnostic test (Fig. 19.5C).

- A diagnostic test with a high specificity (and therefore a low sensitivity) has a low false positive rate (type I error).

Reducing the threshold (by shifting the vertical line to the left) increases the sensitivity but decreases the specificity of the diagnostic test (Fig. 19.5D).

- A diagnostic test with a high sensitivity (and therefore a low specificity) has a low false negative rate (type II error).

Table 19.2 Table of frequencies for a diagnostic test.

		Disease status (according to gold standard test)	
		Disease (positive)	No disease (negative)
Test result	Positive	True positive	False positive (type I error)
	Negative	False negative (type II error)	True negative

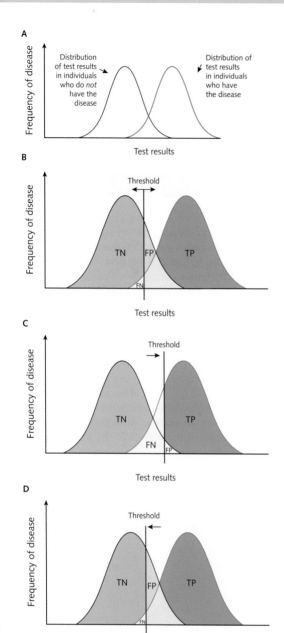

Fig. 19.5 Distribution curve: sensitivity and specificity (see text). *FN, false negative; FP, false positive; TN, true negative; TP, true positive.*

Using sensitivity and specificity to make clinical decisions

As mentioned above, we gain sensitivity at the expense of specificity, and vice versa. Whether we decide to aim for a diagnostic test that has high sensitivity or high specificity (i.e., by decreasing or increasing the threshold, respectively) depends on:

- the condition we are trying to diagnose
- the implications for the patient of either a false negative or false positive test result.

A high sensitivity test is preferred if:

- the disease is life threatening if left untreated
- there is an improvement in survival rate if treatment is initiated early
- overdiagnosis is okay (if a screening test) because all those who screen positive will have further tests.

For example, the absence of retinal vein pulsation for diagnosing raised intracranial pressure, or screening programmes, such as for breast cancer or HIV.
A high specificity test is preferred if:

- the disease is *not* life threatening if left untreated
- subsequent tests or treatments are invasive (e.g., prostate biopsy) or have severe side effects (e.g., chemotherapy)
- treatment costs are high
- the pretest probability of the condition is low.

For example, screening tests for Down syndrome during pregnancy are highly specific, as the consequence of a wrong diagnosis is abortion.

False positives and false negatives

A false negative (type II error) is when an individual is incorrectly diagnosed as not having the disease, when in fact the person does have the disease. If you know the sensitivity of the test, the false negative rate is equal to:

$$\text{False negative}\,(\%) = 100\% - \text{Sensitivity}\,(\%)$$

A false positive (type I error) is when an individual is incorrectly diagnosed as having the disease, when in fact the person is disease free. If you know the specificity of the test, the false positive rate is equal to:

$$\text{False positive}\,(\%) = 100\% - \text{Specificity}\,(\%)$$

Positive and negative predictive values

The sensitivity and specificity are both characteristics of a diagnostic test, but they don't inform us on how to interpret the results of the test for an individual patient. Therefore, in the clinical setting, we use PPV and NPV to indicate the probability that the patient has (or does not have) the disease, given a positive (or negative) test result.

The PPV can be written as:

$$PPV = \frac{\text{True positive}}{\text{True positive} + \text{False positive}}$$
$$= \frac{TP}{TP + FP}$$

A test with a high PPV means that there is only a small percent of false positives within all the individuals with positive test results; i.e., the patient probably does have the disease.

The NPV can be written as:

$$NPV = \frac{\text{True negative}}{\text{True negative} + \text{False negative}}$$
$$= \frac{TN}{TN + FN}$$

A test with a high NPV means that there is only a small percent of false negatives within all the individuals with negative test results; i.e., the patient probably does not have the disease.

COMMON PITFALLS

While the sensitivity and specificity are prevalence-independent tests, predictive values are dependent on the prevalence of the disease in the population being studied.

HINTS AND TIPS

NUMBER NEEDED TO TEST

Another way of expressing the positive predictive value (PPV) is the number needed to test (NNTest). This is the number of patients with a specific symptom who would need to be tested in order to find one true positive. It is calculated as 1/PPV. For instance, if a patient presents in primary care with a new headache that is severe and of sudden onset, the PPV of that history for subarachnoid haemorrhage (SAH) is 25%. The NNTest is therefore 4 – only 4 such patients need to be tested for SAH in order to correctly diagnose one patient with the condition. Patients, and some doctors, find the NNTest easier to understand than the PPV.

THE DIAGNOSTIC PROCESS

The PPV and NPV of a test (or a symptom or sign) are useful measures in clinical practice, especially when a patient wants the clinician to confirm that he doesn't have the disease when the test result is negative. Similarly, a patient may want the clinician to confirm that he definitely has the disease when the test result is positive. When a test is 100% specific, the PPV is 100% as there are never any false-positive results (Fig. 19.6A). When a test is 100% sensitive, the NPV is 100% as there are never any false-negative results (Fig. 19.6B).

Unlike sensitivity and specificity, the PPV and NPV depend on the prevalence of disease in the population (as well as the sensitivity and specificity of the test). In the following section, we will discuss how knowing the disease prevalence in the population can assist us when deciding whether or not to order a particular diagnostic test for your patient.

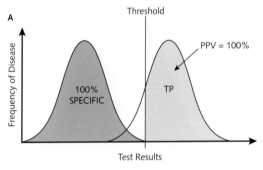

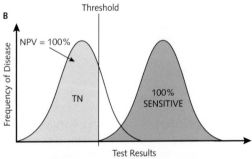

Fig. 19.6 Distribution curve. (A) Positive and (B) negative predictive values. *NPV,* Negative predictive value; *PPV,* positive predictive value; *TN,* true negative; *TP,* true positive.

Case 2: Equivocal pretest probability/high prevalence

A 41-year-old female who has a background of hypertension and smoking presents with a 2-week history of central, stabbing chest pain. It is sometimes precipitated by moderate exertion and there is some costochondral tenderness.

Referring to Table 19.5:

- Her pretest probability of CAD is approximately 50%.
- With a moderate prevalence of 50%, and a relatively high sensitivity and specificity, both the PPV and the NPV are high. Therefore, the results are likely to be correct, whether positive or negative.
- Based on these findings:
  - it is likely that the patient would need an angiogram if the EST result is positive.
  - it is unlikely that the patient would need an angiogram if the EST result is negative; however, as the patient still has a 29% probability (100% – NPV%) of having CAD, an angiogram may be warranted if resources are available and there is enough clinical suspicion.

Case 3: High pretest probability/ high prevalence

A 65-year-old male with a background of hypertension presents with a 6-week history of intermittent central, crushing chest pain that radiates to his jaw. It is usually precipitated by mild exertion and relieved by nitroglycerine or rest.

Referring to Table 19.6:

- His pretest probability of CAD is approximately 90%.
- With a high prevalence of 90% and relatively high sensitivity and specificity, the PPV is high. Therefore, with a PPV of 96%, only 4% of individuals who test positive will not have CAD.
- The NPV is only 21%. Therefore, 79% of individuals who test negative will actually have CAD.
- Overall, if the pretest probability is high, EST doesn't help with clinical decision-making; i.e., with a very high initial pretest probability of 90%, you would perform an angiogram in this patient anyway.

Table 19.5 The effect of moderate prevalence on the predictive value.

		Coronary artery disease (according to gold standard test)		
		Disease (positive)	Disease (negative)	Total
Exercise stress test	Positive	340	115	455
	Negative	160	385	545
	Total	500	500	1000

Sensitivity	340/500 = 68%	PPV	340/455 = 75%
Specificity	385/500 = 77%	NPV	385/545 = 71 %
Prevalence	500/1000 = 50%		

NPV, Negative predictive value; PPV, positive predictive value.

Table 19.6 The effect of high prevalence on the predictive value.

		Coronary artery disease (according to gold standard test)		
		Disease (positive)	Disease (negative)	Total
Exercise stress test	Positive	612	23	635
	Negative	288	77	365
	Total	900	100	1000

Sensitivity	612/900 = 68%	PPV	612/635 = 96%
Specificity	77/100 = 77%	NPV	77/365 = 21%
Prevalence	900/1000 = 90%		

NPV, Negative predictive value; PPV, positive predictive value.

BIAS IN DIAGNOSTIC STUDIES

When assessing the validity of a diagnostic study it is important to consider whether the study design may have been affected by potential biases. For an introduction to study error and bias, please refer to Chapter 12, Bias.

Spectrum bias

Spectrum bias is a type of selection bias that depends on the type of patients recruited for the diagnostic study. It may occur when only cases with a limited range of disease spectrum are recruited for the study.

The performance of a diagnostic test may be artificially overestimated if a case–control study design is used in which healthy volunteers ('fittest of the fit') are compared with a population with advanced disease ('sickest of the sick') (Fig. 19.9A). As demonstrated using the example in the previous section, this diagnostic test will have limited value as these cases have already been diagnosed; i.e., the pretest probability is already very low or very high and the test will make little difference. On the other hand, if the diagnostic study is based on a cohort study design, during which a representative population is evaluated (Fig. 19.9B), there will be less spectrum bias.

The likelihood ratio is not affected by spectrum bias and can be used in case-control studies that separately recruit people with and without the disease.

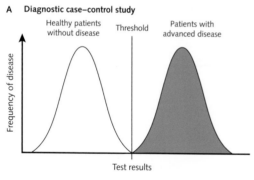

A   Diagnostic case–control study

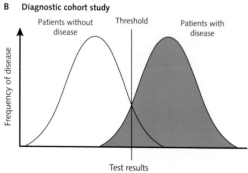

B   Diagnostic cohort study

Fig. 19.9 Spectrum bias: more likely in case–control than in cohort studies. (A) Diagnostic case–control study. (B) Diagnostic cohort study.

Verification bias

Verification bias:

- generally only occurs when patients are tested with the study test before the reference (gold standard) test.
- is a type of nonrandom misclassification measurement bias (discussed in Chapter 12).
- can be divided into:
  - Partial verification bias, or
  - Differential verification bias.

Partial verification bias

Partial verification bias (also known as work-up bias):

- occurs when the decision to perform the reference (gold standard) test on an individual is based on the results of the diagnostic study test. For example, the gold standard test may only be performed on those patients who have a positive study test result. Consequently, more unwell individuals (than healthy ones) undergo gold standard testing. This will lead to an underestimation of the false-negative rate and an overestimation of both the NPV and the sensitivity of the study test. Therefore, if individuals who have negative study test results do not undergo gold standard testing, the diagnostic test would be perceived to be better as the number of positive cases detected would be higher. However, the degree of partial verification bias would also be higher in this situation.
- is usually an issue if the gold standard test is:
  1. invasive, such as surgery or biopsy, and therefore unethical for use in individuals in whom there is very minimal clinical suspicion of disease.
  2. expensive.
- may be an issue if those individuals with a positive study test result undergo a more extended period of follow-up than those individuals with a negative study test result.
- may be avoided if the reference test is always performed prior to the study test. However, this is not always possible; for example, you wouldn't perform surgery prior to imaging.
- may be minimized in some study designs by blinding the investigator between the study test and reference test results.

Differential verification bias

Differential verification bias occurs when different reference tests are used to verify the results of the study test. It may be an issue if patients testing positive on the study test receive a more accurate, often more invasive, reference test than those with negative test results. Therefore, using a less invasive, often less accurate, reference test on those individuals with a negative study test result may lead to an increase in the specificity of the study test.

CHOOSING APPROPRIATE STATISTICAL TESTS

In previous chapters we discussed how to calculate and interpret the different measures of association, including the risk ratio (Chapter 12) and odds ratio (Chapter 13). On some occasions, we compare two competing variables by calculating the difference between the group means (or group proportions) (Chapter 8). We can also calculate the 95% confidence interval for these measures of association to determine how precisely we have determined the differences of interest. It combines the variability (standard deviation) and sample size to generate a confidence interval for the population measure (Chapter 8). We use the measure of association and the confidence interval to put the result in a scientific context. However, we must also determine whether the results obtained are statistically significant by calculating the *P*-value (please refer to Chapter 8 for a discussion on how to interpret the *P*-value).

Having defined the null and alternative hypotheses for your comparison, an appropriate statistical test is used to compute the *P*-value from the sample data. The *P*-value provides a measure of evidence for or against the null hypothesis. If the *P*-value shows evidence against the null hypothesis being tested, then the alternative hypothesis must be true. In some undergraduate curriculums you are expected to know which statistical tests to use (to calculate the *P*-value) when analysing different data sets. Selecting the most appropriate statistical test depends on three key pieces of information:

1. The goal of the data analysis
2. The type of variable you are analysing
3. The distribution of the data.

Data analysis goal

What is the aim of your analysis? Are you:

- comparing one group to a hypothetical value?
- comparing two unpaired groups?
- comparing two paired groups?
- comparing three or more unmatched groups?
- comparing three or more matched groups?
- quantifying the association between two variables?

COMMON PITFALLS

- If the groups are paired (or matched), this implies they are dependent; i.e., repeated measurements of the same variable in the same subject.
- If the groups are unpaired (or unmatched), this implies they are independent; i.e., the same variable is measured in two different groups of subjects.

COMMON PITFALLS

It can sometimes be difficult to distinguish between an interval and ratio variable. For the purpose of choosing an appropriate statistical test for your data, it is important to only identify whether your data is numerical or not.

Type of variable

It is important to define the type of variable you are analysing.

- Research data usually fall into one of the four types of variables:
- Nominal ⎱
- Ordinal ⎰ Categorical variable
- Interval ⎱
- Ratio ⎰ Numerical variable

Please refer to Chapter 7 for a discussion on these different types of variables.

Data distribution

Gaussian versus non-Gaussian distributions

Choosing the right statistical test to compare measurements also depends on the distribution of the data. There is no need to check the distribution of the data when dealing with nominal or ordinal variables. The distribution of the data should only be checked for interval or ratio variables. Statistical tests based upon the assumption that the data are sampled from a Gaussian (or normal) distribution are referred to as parametric tests. Some parametric tests also assume that the variance (or standard deviation) is equal in all groups being compared. Statistical tests that do not assume that the data follow a Gaussian distribution are referred to as nonparametric tests. Commonly used nonparametric tests involve ranking the outcome variable values from low to high and then analysing the distribution of the ranks.

When to choose a nonparametric test

Formal statistical tests, such as the D'Agostino–Pearson test or the Kolmogorov–Smirnov test, are frequently used to check the distribution of the data. The null hypothesis of these tests (known as normality tests) state that the data are taken from a population that follows a Gaussian (normal) distribution. If the P-value is low, demonstrating that the data do not follow a Gaussian distribution, a nonparametric test is usually chosen. However, normality tests should not be used to automatically decide whether to use a nonparametric test or not. While the normality test can assist you in making your decision, the following considerations should also be made:

- If your data do not follow a Gaussian distribution (i.e., the distribution is skewed), consider transforming the data, perhaps using reciprocals or logarithms, to convert non-Gaussian data to a Gaussian distribution (discussed in Chapter 7). The data can subsequently be analysed using a parametric statistical test.
- The results from a single normality test should be interpreted in context. This is usually an issue if additional data from another experiment need to be analysed in the same way. Consequently, you cannot rely on the results from a single normality test.

- Whether or not to choose a nonparametric test matters the most when the samples are small.

On some occasions, you may decide to use a nonparametric test if, in addition to the data not having a Gaussian distribution, the variances are not equal between the groups being compared. Considering skewness and differences in variances often coexist, correcting for one (e.g., by transforming the data) may also correct the other. However, some parametric tests can still be used if they are adjusted to take account of these unequal variances.

Sample size matters

When the sample size is small (e.g., $n < 15$):

- parametric tests are not very robust when analysing data that do not follow a Gaussian distribution.
- nonparametric tests have little power to detect a significant difference when analysing data that follow a Gaussian distribution (please refer to Chapter 8 for a discussion on statistical power).
- you are likely to get a high P-value when using a nonparametric test to analyse data that follow a Gaussian distribution.
- normality tests have little power to detect whether a sample comes from a Gaussian distribution.

When the sample size is large (e.g., $n > 100$):

- parametric tests are robust when analysing data that do not follow a Gaussian distribution.
- nonparametric tests almost have as much power as parametric tests when analysing data that follow a Gaussian distribution.
- normality tests have high power to detect whether or not a sample comes from a Gaussian distribution.

Table 20.1 summarizes the implications of sample size when interpreting the results of parametric, nonparametric and normality tests.

Table 20.1 The effect of sample size on statistical testing.

	Small sample size	Large sample size
Using parametric tests on data with a non-Gaussian distribution	Not very robust – may produce misleading results	Robust
Using nonparametric tests on data with a Gaussian distribution	Little power – may produce misleading results	Almost have as much power as parametric tests
Normality test (e.g., D'Agostino–Pearson test)	Low power for detecting whether or not a sample comes from a Gaussian distribution	High power for detecting whether or not a sample comes from a Gaussian distribution

When dealing with large sample sizes, the decision to choose a parametric or nonparametric test matters less.

HINTS AND TIPS

DATA ANALYSIS

You can access online calculators, which will assist you in calculating a number of the statistical tests outlined in this chapter. GraphPad have an online version of their statistical package that can be accessed at http://www.graphpad.com/quickcalcs/

COMPARISON OF ONE GROUP TO A HYPOTHETICAL VALUE

When the primary aim of your analysis is to compare one group to a hypothetical value, the flowchart in Fig. 20.1

should be followed to identify the most suitable statistical test for your data.

COMPARISON OF TWO GROUPS

When the primary aim of your analysis is to compare two groups, the flowchart in Fig. 20.2 should be followed to identify the most suitable statistical test for your data.

Chi-square test and Fisher exact test

The chi-square test and Fisher exact test compare the proportions of outcomes in different groups. In other words, they test for an association between two categorical variables. The data are obtained, initially, as 'observed' frequencies; i.e., the numbers with and without the outcome in each of the two groups (exposed and unexposed) being compared. These frequencies can be entered into a contingency table. If the table has two rows and two columns, it is known as a 2×2 contingency table (Table 20.2). For an example of a contingency table used as part of a study, please refer to Chapter 13, Fig. 13.4. We can subsequently calculate the frequency that we would expect in each of the four cells of the contingency table if the null hypothesis were true. These are known as the 'expected' ('E') frequencies (Table 20.3).

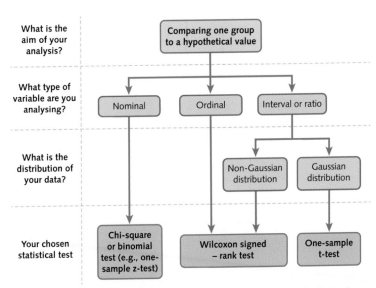

Fig. 20.1 Flowchart for selection of statistical tests comparing one group with a hypothetical value.

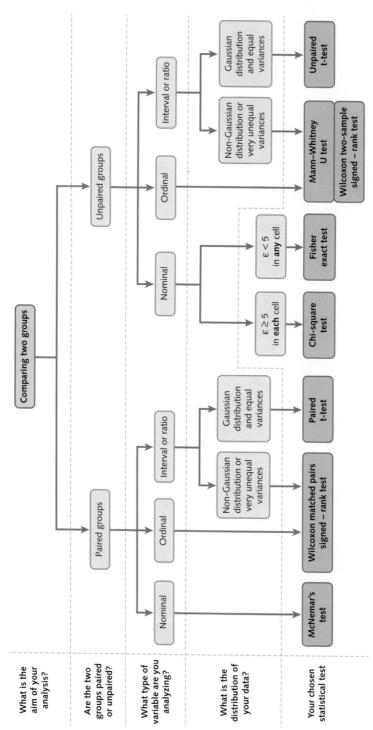

Fig. 20.2 Flowchart for selection of statistical tests comparing two groups.

- Were individuals lost to follow up? If yes, did individuals lost to follow up differ systematically from those who remained in the study?
- Is the disease status of the tested population clearly defined? If only cases with a limited range of disease spectrum are recruited for the study, there is potential for spectrum bias.
- Was there an independent, blind comparison between the diagnostic test and the reference gold standard test? Partial verification bias (also known as work-up bias) may occur when the decision to perform the reference gold standard test on an individual is based on the results of the diagnostic test.
- Were the methods used for performing the test described in sufficient detail? A protocol should be followed. Differential verification bias may occur when different reference tests are used to verify the results of the study diagnostic test.
- Are all the test characteristics presented? The accuracy (sensitivity and specificity) and performance (positive and negative predictive values) of the test should be reported. Confidence intervals should be provided for these measures.
- Could interpretation of the results of the diagnostic test have been influenced by knowledge of the results of the reference standard test, and vice versa? Reporting bias may be an issue if there is a degree of subjectivity in interpreting the results.
- Were the methods for performing the test described in sufficient detail to permit replication?
- Have the study findings regarding the accuracy and performance of the diagnostic test been placed in the wider context of other (potential) tests in the diagnostic process?
- How do the results fit in locally? Does your local setting differ much from that of the study?
- Can the diagnostic test be applied to your patient (or population) of interest? The following should be considered:
  - opportunity costs
  - level of expertise required to perform the test and interpret the results
  - number of resources available
  - availability of services.
- What impact would the test have if used in your local setting? This may include implications for patient management or healthcare costs.

CRITICAL APPRAISAL CHECKLIST: QUALITATIVE STUDIES

- Does the qualitative study ask a clearly defined, well-focused and clinically important question?
- Was it appropriate to answer this question using a qualitative study design?
- Do the study investigators explain how potential participants were selected? Why were these participants chosen in particular?
- What sampling strategy was used to address the study aims; i.e., purposive sampling, quota sampling, snowball sampling, etc.? Was this the most appropriate sampling strategy to address the study aims? Are there any major limitations to the sampling strategy?
- What methods were used for data collection; i.e., participant observation, in-depth interviews or focus groups? Was this the most suitable method of data collection? Was the data collected at the most appropriate setting; e.g., the participant's own home, at a clinic, etc.?
- What was the investigator's perspective and how did this influence (or bias) data collection; i.e., reflexivity?
- Is there any evidence of triangulation?
- Were the study findings well 'grounded' in the data? Was the constant comparison approach used to clarify emerging themes?
- Is there any evidence of iteration between data collection and analysis?
- Did the investigators continue until they reached data saturation?
- Were all data collected taken into account? For example, did the investigators include data on negative cases; i.e., those against the emerging theme?
- Was sufficient raw data included in the final report to enable the reader to draw the same conclusions as the study investigators?
- Would another researcher be able to reproduce the same data and interpret it in the same way? To assess for interrater reliability, did a second investigator independently code the data?
- What was the main study finding? Are the conclusions drawn justified by the findings?
- Are the findings applicable (or transferrable) to other patients and/or settings? There should be a detailed description of the context and setting in which the study was undertaken.
- Are the findings of this study likely to have any relevance for clinical practice

Chapter Summary

- Critical appraisal is the process of systematically examining the available evidence to judge its validity, results and relevance in a particular context.
- It is important to determine both the internal validity and external validity of the study you are appraising.
- External validity refers to the extent to which the study findings are generalizable beyond the limits of the study to the study's target population.
- Internal validity ensures that the study was run carefully (research design, how variables were measured, etc.) and the extent to which the observed effect(s) were produced solely by the intervention being assessed (and not by another factor).
- A number of key points, including potential confounding factors and sources of selection/measurement bias, should be reviewed when appraising all research papers regardless of the study design employed.
- There are specific critical appraisal checklists for more complex study designs, including systematic reviews (and meta-analyses), randomized controlled trials, diagnostic studies and qualitative studies.

FURTHER READING

Delgado-Rodríguez, M., Bias, L.J., 2004. J. Epidemiol Community Health 58, 635–641.

Greenhalgh, T., 2014. How to Read a Paper: The Basics of Evidence-Based Medicine, fifth ed. Wiley-Blackwell, London.

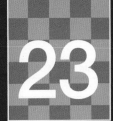
The application of the formulae listed in this chapter will be expected in most evidence-based medicine undergraduate and postgraduate exams. Furthermore, some medical schools and exam bodies expect you to memorize these formulae as they may not be provided in the exam. Please refer to the respective chapters for a more in-depth discussion about each of the formulae listed.

DESCRIBING THE FREQUENCY DISTRIBUTION

We can summarize the data (or frequency distribution) of a variable using the formulae listed in Table 23.1. The formulae listed in Table 23.1 are covered in Chapter 7 of this book.

EXTRAPOLATING FROM 'SAMPLE' TO 'POPULATION'

Having chosen an appropriate study sample, the rules of probability are applied to make inferences about the overall population from which the sample was drawn (Table 23.2). The formulae used to make this inference depend on whether you are dealing with:

- a single group mean
- a single group proportion
- two independent means
- paired means
- two independent proportions.

The formulae listed in Table 23.2 are covered in Chapter 7 of this book.

STUDY ANALYSIS

Different formulae are used when analysing the results from different study designs (Table 23.3), including:

Table 23.1 Formulae used to describe the frequency distribution

	Formula	Key
Arithmetic mean $\bar{x}$ (x – bar)	$\bar{x} = \dfrac{x_1 + x_2 + x_3 + \cdots + x_n}{n}$ $\bar{x} = \dfrac{\sum_{i=1}^{n} x_i}{n}$	• x = variable • n = number of observations of the variable • Σ (sigma) = the sum of (the observations of the variable) • Sub- and superscripts on the Σ = sum of the observations from $i = 1$ to n NOTE: The arithmetic mean of a population is denoted using the symbol μ.
Population variance σ^2	$\sigma^2 = \dfrac{\Sigma(x_i - \bar{x})^2}{n}$	• x = variable • $\bar{x}$ (x – bar) = mean of the variable x • x_i = individual observation • n = number of observations of the variable • Σ (sigma) = the sum of (the squared differences of the individual observations from the mean)
Population standard deviation σ	$\sigma = \sqrt{\sigma^2}$	• σ^2 = population variance
Sample variance s^2	$s^2 = \dfrac{\Sigma(x_i - \bar{x})^2}{n-1}$	The symbols are identical to those used for the population variance
Sample standard deviation s	$s = \sqrt{s^2}$	• s^2 = sample variance
95% reference range	mean $- [1.96 \times \text{SD(mean)}]$ to mean $+ [1.96 \times \text{SD(mean)}]$	• SD(mean) = standard deviation of the mean NOTE: The equation is the same whether you are calculating the 95% reference range for sample or population data

Table 23.2 Formulae used when extrapolating data from sample to population

	Formula	Key
Standard error of a single mean (SEM)	$SEM = \dfrac{SD}{\sqrt{n}}$	• SD = standard deviation • n = number of observations
95% Confidence interval for a single mean	mean $- [1.96 \times SE(\text{mean})]$ to mean $+ [1.96 \times SE(\text{mean})]$	• SE(mean) = standard error of the mean NOTE: This equation only applies for large samples
Standard error of a single proportion SE(p)	$SE(p) = \sqrt{\dfrac{p \times (1-p)}{n}}$	• p = proportion • n = number of observations
95% Confidence interval for a single proportion	proportion $- [1.96 \times SE(p)]$ to proportion $+ [1.96 \times SE(p)]$	• SE(p) = standard error of the proportion NOTE: This equation only applies for large samples
Standard error of difference between two independent means $SE(\bar{x}_1 - \bar{x}_0)$	$SE(\bar{x}_1 - \bar{x}_0) = \sqrt{\left[SE(\bar{x}_1)\right]^2 + \left[SE(\bar{x}_0)\right]^2}$	• $SE(\bar{x}_1)$ = standard error of mean of group 1 • $SE(\bar{x}_0)$ = standard error of mean of group 0
95% Confidence interval for the difference between two independent means	95% CI for $(\bar{x}_1 - \bar{x}_0) =$ $(\bar{x}_1 - \bar{x}_0) - \left[1.96 \times SE(\bar{x}_1 - \bar{x}_0)\right]$ to $(\bar{x}_1 - \bar{x}_0) + \left[1.96 \times SE(\bar{x}_1 - \bar{x}_0)\right]$	• $(\bar{x}_1 - \bar{x}_0)$ = difference in means between two independent groups, group 0 and group 1 • $SE(\bar{x}_1 - \bar{x}_0)$ = standard error of the difference in means between group 0 and group 1
Standard error of the difference between paired means $SE(\bar{d})$	$SE(\bar{d}) = \dfrac{SD(d)}{\sqrt{n}}$	• SD(d) = standard deviation of the difference between all paired observations • n = number of paired observations
95% Confidence interval for the difference between paired means	95% CI$(\bar{d}) = \bar{d} - \left[1.96 \times SE(\bar{d})\right]$ to $\bar{d} + \left[1.96 \times SE(\bar{d})\right]$	• $\bar{d}$ = mean of paired differences • $SE(\bar{d})$ = standard error of mean of paired differences
Standard error of the difference between two independent proportions SE(p1 − p0)	$SE(p_1 - p_0) = \sqrt{SE(p_1)^2 + SE(p_0)^2}$	• SE(p1) = standard error of proportion of group 1 • SE(p0) = standard error of proportion of group 0
95% Confidence interval for the difference between two independent proportions	95% CI for (p1 − p0) = (p1 − p0) $- [1.96 \times SE(p1 - p0)]$ to (p1 − p0) $+ [1.96 \times SE(p1 - p0)]$	• (p1 − p0) = difference in proportions between group 1 and group 0 • SE(p1 − p0) = standard error of difference in proportions between group 1 and group 0

CI, confidence interval

Table 23.3 Analysing study data

Study	Formula
Randomized controlled trial	
Number needed to treat to benefit (NNTB) or number needed to treat to harm (NNTH)	$NNTB \text{ or } NNTH = \dfrac{1}{|\text{Risk difference between two treatment groups}|}$
Cohort study	
Incidence of disease	Incidence risk $= \dfrac{\text{Number of new cases of the disease in a given time period}}{\text{Total number of subjects initially disease free}}$ Incidence rate $= \dfrac{\text{Number of new cases of the disease in a given time period}}{\text{Total number of subjects initially disease free} \times \text{Time interval}}$
Risk ratio (RR)	$RR = \dfrac{\text{Risk in exposed group}}{\text{Risk in unexposed group}}$
Risk difference (RD)	RD = Risk in exposed group − Risk in unexposed group

Table 23.3 Analysing study data—cont'd

Study	Formula
Case–control study	
Odds of exposure	$\text{Odds of exposure} = \dfrac{\text{Probability of being exposed}}{\text{Probability of being unexposed}}$
Exposure odds ratio (OR)	$\text{Exposure OR} = \dfrac{\text{Odds of exposure in cases}}{\text{Odds of exposure in controls}}$
Odds of disease	$\text{Odds of disease} = \dfrac{\text{Probability of having disease}}{\text{Probability of not having disease}}$
Disease OR	$\text{Disease OR} = \dfrac{\text{Odds of disease amongst exposed subjects}}{\text{Odds of disease amongst unexposed subjects}}$
Cross-sectional study	
Prevalence	$\text{Prevalence} = \dfrac{\text{Number of new and old cases of the disease at a single point in time}}{\text{Total number of people in the population at the same point in time}}$
Prevalence OR	$\text{Prevalence OR} = \dfrac{\text{Odds of the disease amongst the exposed subjects at a single point in time}}{\text{Odds of the disease amongst the unexposed subjects at the same point in time}}$
Prevalence ratio	$\text{Prevalence ratio} = \dfrac{\text{Probability of the disease amongst the exposed subjects at a single point in time}}{\text{Probability of the disease amongst the unexposed subjects at the same point in time}}$

- randomized controlled trials
- cohort studies
- case–control studies
- cross-sectional studies.

Please refer to the relevant study design chapter for an in-depth discussion on how to apply each formula to sample data.

TEST PERFORMANCE

As clinicians, we rely on diagnostic tests to make decisions on how we treat our patients. Therefore, the performance (or validity) of a new test must be properly assessed before implementing its use in the clinical setting (Table 23.4). The formulae listed in Table 23.4 are covered in Chapter 19 of this book.

Table 23.4 Analysing the performance of a test

Measure of test performance	Formula
False positive (FP) rate	$FP(\%) = 100\% - \text{Specificity (\%)}$
False negative (FN) rate	$FN(\%) = 100\% - \text{Sensitivity (\%)}$
Sensitivity	$\text{Sensitivity} = \dfrac{\text{True positive}}{\text{True positive} + \text{False negative}}$
Specificity	$\text{Specificity} = \dfrac{\text{True negative}}{\text{True negative} + \text{False positive}}$
Positive predictive value (PPV)	$PPV = \dfrac{\text{True positive}}{\text{True positive} + \text{False positive}}$
Negative predictive value (NPV)	$NPV = \dfrac{\text{True negative}}{\text{True negative} + \text{False negative}}$
Positive likelihood ratio (LR+)	$LR+ = \dfrac{\text{Sensitivity}}{1 - \text{Specificity}}$
Negative likelihood ratio (LR−)	$LR- = \dfrac{1 - \text{Sensitivity}}{\text{Specificity}}$

Table 23.5 Economic evaluation

Economic Measure		Formula
Cost-utility analysis	Utility score	$\text{Utility score} = \dfrac{\text{Number of years alive at full health}}{\text{Number of years alive at poorer health state}}$
	Quality-adjusted life year (QALY)	QALY = Period of time spent in a health state × Utility score for that health state
	Incremental cost-effectiveness ratio (ICER)	$\text{ICER} = \dfrac{\text{Cost of intervention A} - \text{Cost of intervention B}}{\text{Number of QALYs for intervention A} - \text{Number of QALYs for intervention B}}$
	Net monetary benefit (NMB)	NMB = [(Number of QALYs for intervention A − Number of QALYs for intervention B) × λ] − (Cost of intervention A − Cost of intervention B)
		where λ is the amount that society is willing to pay per QALY
Cost-effectiveness analysis	Cost-effectiveness ratio (CER)	$\text{Cost effectiveness ratio} = \dfrac{\text{Cost of intervention}}{\text{Health effect outcome}}$
	ICER	$\text{ICER} = \dfrac{\text{Cost of intervention A} - \text{Cost of intervention B}}{\text{Health effects of intervention A} - \text{Health effects of intervention B}}$

ECONOMIC EVALUATION

A full economic evaluation of healthcare involves systematically comparing the costs (inputs) and benefits (outcomes) of at least two alternative interventions to evaluate the best use of the scarce resources available. Some of the key formulae used to evaluate the cost effectiveness of competing interventions are covered in Table 23.5. The formulae listed in Table 23.5 are covered in Chapter 21 of this book.

FURTHER READING

Bland, M., 2015. An Introduction to Medical Statistics, second ed. Oxford University Press, Oxford.

Motulsky, H.J. GraphPad Statistics Guide. Available from: https://www.graphpad.com/guides/prism/7/statistics/index.htm [Accessed 21st September 2018].

Motulsky, H.J., 2017. Intuitive Biostatistics: A Nonmathematical Guide to Statistical Thinking, fourth ed. Oxford University Press, Oxford.

AUDIT AND ITS LOOP: THE MODERN APPROACH TO IMPROVING HEALTH-CARE PRACTICE

Chapter 24

Clinical audit 227

Chapter 25

Quality improvement 235

AN INTRODUCTION TO CLINICAL AUDIT

Clinical governance

There is public and professional belief in the provision of high-quality care that is not only effective but also safe. Clinical governance is the systematic approach used to maintain and improve the quality of patient care within a health system. Key areas of clinical governance include:

- research
- education and training
- clinical audit
- clinical effectiveness.

What is clinical audit?

Clinical audit is at the heart of clinical governance, reviewing the quality of current practice against explicit criteria of expected healthcare standards. The audit process is usually represented by a cycle, which emphasizes its ongoing nature (Fig. 24.1). Audits use a systematic approach to confirm the quality of clinical services, highlighting the need for quality improvement (at an individual, team or service level) where necessary. However, how do we define high-quality care? How do we determine what best practice is? The answer to both these questions, in addition to life's many mysteries, is research!

Clinical audit versus clinical research

The key difference between audit and research is in the aim of the study. While clinical research aims to establish what is the best or most effective practice, clinical audit evaluates how closely local practice resembles this. Audits may generate new research questions, which may subsequently be investigated using a research protocol. Audit and research may therefore follow each other in a cycle (Fig. 24.2). There may be a number of audit cycles prior to identifying an important or relevant question, if any.

Similarities between audit and research

With fundamental goals of improving healthcare, a number of similarities exist between audit and research. They both:

- address an important question related to clinical practice.
- involve writing protocols, specifying the appropriate type and size of sample.
- collect necessary information required to answer the question.
- involve analysing the data collected and interpreting the results.
- involve sharing the results in order to promote healthcare change.

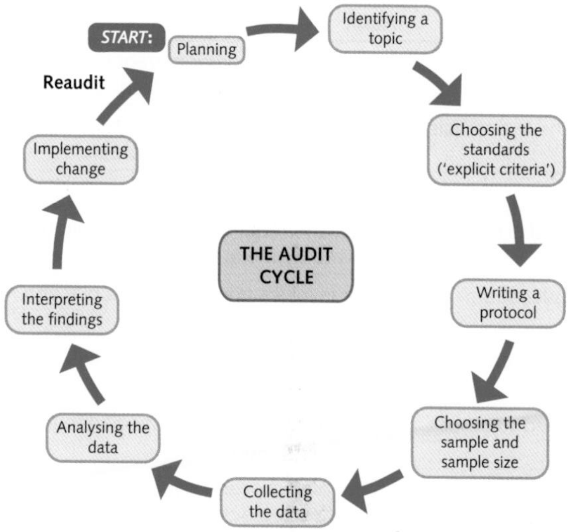

Fig. 24.1 The audit cycle.

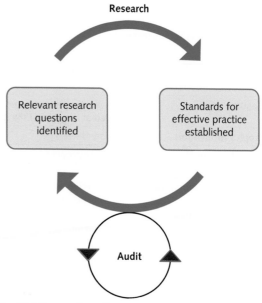

Fig. 24.2 Research–audit cycle.

Differences between audit and research

It is sometimes difficult to distinguish between audit and research, or decide whether an audit or research study is required to answer your question. Table 24.1 summarizes the key differences between clinical audit and clinical research.

HINTS AND TIPS

As healthcare professionals, it is important that we not only understand the principles and methodology of the audit process, but that we undertake our own audit projects under appropriate guidance and supervision. Participating in clinical audit forms a routine part of clinical training and practice.

PLANNING THE AUDIT

Prior to starting the audit project, it is important to:

- ensure you have enough time to plan and complete the audit cycle prior to starting.
- identify a supervisor or relevant clinical lead in whom you can rely upon for advice and support.
- make yourself known to the local audit department, who will advise you on data protection and confidentiality issues.
- consider whether you will need support in collecting data.

HINTS AND TIPS

When setting up your audit, key staff and committee members should be identified in your organization:

- Clinical audit manager (the operational lead for the clinical audit)
- Designated clinical lead and facilitators in your clinical division or directorate
- Clinical audit committee (they have responsibility for overseeing clinical audit practice)
- The team responsible for providing and coordinating clinical audit training.

Identifying a topic

Sources of inspiration

Even if you decide to carry out your audit project independently, it is important to involve stakeholders who have an involvement in the health service when deciding on potential topics. Stakeholders may include:

- patients
- clinicians
- medical records personnel
- audit department staff.

The audit question may be based on your clinical experience. For example:

- when new clinical guidelines have been implemented into practice (based on research evidence) and you want to audit how well they have been introduced.

Table 24.1 Audit versus research.

	Research	Audit
Aims	To establish what best practice is	To determine whether current local practice resembles best practice
Results	The results are compared with the hypothesis stated at the start of the study	The results are compared with standards that define best practice
Project motivation	Theory driven	Practice based
Ethical approval	Formal ethical review and approval is required	Not always required (project should be reviewed by the audit department)
Treatment administration	May involve administration of a placebo or a completely novel treatment	Never involves administering a placebo or a novel treatment
Random allocation	Patient groups may be randomly allocated to different interventions	Never involves randomly allocating patients to different interventions
Generalizability of findings	Yes—the results can be generalized to other similar group or populations	No—the results are only specific to the local patient group audited
After completing the project?	An ongoing process involving investigation of *new* research questions with every project	An ongoing process involving a number of audit cycles evaluating the *same* clinical standards

- when you feel there is variation in healthcare practice between different wards at the same hospital.
- in areas where there is a high risk to the patients, staff or the organization.
- in areas involving high-cost interventions.

It is important to perform a literature search and consider the findings of recently published reviews to identify those areas where clinical practice could be improved. Other *simpler* ways of identifying an appropriate audit question may include:

- looking at already prepared tools; for example, using templates provided by the National Institute for Clinical Excellence that audit the implementation of their clinical guidelines.
- asking the audit department whether they have any audits scheduled to be repeated or whether they have already identified a list of relevant audit questions (sometimes based on local priorities).
- looking for protocols used in the department that performance could be audited against.

Formulating the audit question

Having decided which area of healthcare you wish to audit, is important to formulate a specific question that may address one of the following:

- An outcome, such as cost effectiveness, patient satisfaction, quality of life, survival, infection or readmission rates.
- A process, which refers to protocols, such as involving follow up, team handovers or whether, for example, the troponin level was measured in patients presenting with central chest pain.
- A structure, which refers to the resources available, including the number of patient beds on a ward and the current knowledge, skills and attitudes of the staff.

It is important to define the overall purpose of the project at its start, stating why the audit is being carried out and what it intends to achieve. You are unlikely to deliver full impact without a clear audit question or objective.

CHOOSING THE STANDARDS

Current clinical practice should be compared to a defined set of 'explicit criteria' that:

- reflect best practice.
- are evidence based.
- focus on key parts of the care pathway.
- cover the different aspects of service, including the structure, process and outcome of care.
- must be measurable.

The *standards* define the threshold of the expected performance for each criterion. They are usually expressed as a percentage, for example:

- you expect criterion 1 to be achieved by 100% of the cases audited. This may represent the performance level of the top 5% in the region.
- you expect criterion 1 to be achieved by 90% of the cases audited. This may represent an average performance level.

Choosing the appropriate level of performance that you are trying to achieve is known as 'benchmarking'.

> **HINTS AND TIPS**
>
> If the level of care is measured without comparing the performance to a defined standard, this is known as a service evaluation.

AUDIT PROTOCOL

Having already identified a topic of interest, defined the audit criteria and chosen the benchmark for your standards, a protocol that provides enough detail to allow someone to repeat the audit at a later date needs to be prepared. It should describe the various steps of the audit cycle from start to finish. In addition to helping to ensure that the project is on track, it will allow potential problems to be identified and addressed before they occur. The following points should be outlined in your protocol:

- Title of audit project.
- Background information, describing the clinical setting and the importance of the topic selected.
- The audit question.
- A definition of the explicit criteria.
- A definition of the sample type and how sample size will be determined.
- A description of what information will be required and how will it be collected.
  - Will administrative staff need to pull patient notes?
  - Are the data available electronically?
- A design for the data collection form.
- How will the data be analysed?
- A plan to draw conclusions and make appropriate recommendations.
  - Will the results need to be compared to previous audit results?
- How will the findings be disseminated?
- A plan to repeat the audit cycle to ensure any changes have been made.
- What is your timeline for all steps of the audit cycle?

Your supervisor or clinical lead should review a draft copy of the audit protocol. The feedback received should be considered and amendments made to the protocol, if necessary.

DEFINING THE SAMPLE

A detailed account outlining which patients are eligible for your audit should be discussed. The sampling frame should be described in terms of:

- Sampling method
  - Random sampling: For example, each patient in the chosen setting has an equal probability of selection; eligible patients are allocated a number and a random number generator is used to identify your sample.
  - *Consecutive sampling*: For example, the first patient is randomly selected, then patients consecutively admitted are selected until the required sample size is achieved.
- Sample size
  - This will depend on:
    - resource constraints, such as costs and the number of hours you can afford to invest for data collection prior to your deadline.
    - the degree of confidence you want in your findings.
  - There is often a compromise between the statistical validity of the results and the practical issues associated with data collection.
- Person
  - Demographic profile, i.e., age range or sex?
  - A particular group of patients, i.e., those with a particular diagnosis or who are having a particular intervention?
- Place
  - Primary care?
  - Hospital ward?

- Inpatient or outpatient clinic?
- Health authority?
- Time
  - Depending on the resources available and the admission rate, what are the starting and predicted finishing dates for data collection?
  - Are samples going to be chosen prospectively or retrospectively (Table 24.2)?

DATA COLLECTION

The data may be collected from various sources, including:

- paper medical records
- electronic medical records
- disease registries.

The data collected should:

- be valid by ensuring that it relates directly to the agreed objectives and audit criteria.
- be reliable by ensuring that the same (or almost the same) judgements about performance are made at different times and by different people.
- comply with the accepted ethical principles.
- be consistent with the accepted confidentiality principles by ensuring patient and staff identities are not revealed (identifiable information should not be used).

A paper data collection form or template should be designed that includes very precise definitions of the variables that need to be filled out for each subject. The data collection form should be piloted to ensure that the information collected is:

- informed by the audit criteria.
- consistent.
- comparable between cases.
- kept at a minimum.

Table 24.2 Retrospective versus prospective sampling.

	Retrospective	Prospective
Data collection	Involves reviewing previously collected information about the patient	Data are collected from new admissions
Data source	Routinely documented patient information is used. Adequate sources of retrospective data may not exist	Within the remit of the audit criteria, additional information can be collected to what is routinely documented for the patient
Resources	Less resources (cost, time, manpower) are required to collect the data	More resources are usually required to collect the data
Measurement bias	Less prone to measurement bias: as information has already been collected, the data reviewed are a snapshot of the level of performance at that time	More prone to measurement bias: normal practice may change if people are aware that their performance is being audited

Table 25.2 Patient summary and handover proforma.

Location	Details	Current Admission	Comorbidities	Operation/ Radiology	Social Issues	Current Issues	Management Plan	Key Blood Results
Bed 1	Patient name: Rina Kaura Date of birth: 08/02/1922 Hospital number: 111 1111 111	Presenting complaint: Shortness of breath Diagnosis: LRTI Atrial flutter → T2RF→BiPAP	1) T2DM 2) MI – 09/11 3) AF – on warfarin 4) HTN 5) Hypothyroid	Echo – mild LV impairment LVH ∆ cor pulmonale X-ray Rt Shoulder: loss of rotator cuff tendon, degenerative changes	Lives alone Carer's BD	1) Peripheral oedema 2) Pain/↓ROM right shoulder 3) Reduced mobility 4) LRTI	Medical: Physiotherapy OT Fluid management on co-trimoxazole until 19/02/12 Discharge plan:	ANA +'ve (28/02/12) CRP 52 (27/02/12)

Jobs:

Patient name and bed	Additional relevant medical details	Out-of-hours job	HO	SHO
Rina Kaura Bed 1	Patient on co-trimoxazole for LRTI – possible interaction with warfarin	Patient has atrial fibrillation Please prescribe warfarin	X	

AF, atrial fibrillation; ANA, anti-nuclear antibody; BD, twice-daily; BiPAP, Bilevel Positive Airway Pressure; CRP, C-reactive protein; Echo, echocardiography; HTN, hypertension; HO, house officer; LRTI, lower respiratory tract infection; LV, left ventricular; LVH, left ventricular hypertrophy; MI, myocardial infarction; OT, occupational therapy; ROM, range of motion; Rt, right; SHO, senior house officer; T2DM, type 2 diabetes mellitus; T2RF, type 2 respiratory failure.

Patient summary proforma (standardized ward list)

1. Bed number
2. Demographic information
3. Presenting complaint and diagnosis
4. Comorbidities
5. Operations/procedures
6. Current issues
7. Management plan
8. Discharge plan and social issues
9. Key blood results
10. Jobs

Patient handover proforma

1. Patient name and bed number
2. Additional relevant medical details
3. Out-of-hours jobs
4. Job for completion by: house officer (HO) or senior house officer (SHO)

- All doctors would be informed of the pilot handover system via trust email.
- The initial rounds of data collection would be carried out on the Care of the Elderly ward.
- The day-based ward doctors would electronically complete the patient summary and handover proforma, and subsequently print out hard copies for the out-of-hours doctors.
- Additionally, the on-call team would have access to the proforma via the trust intranet.
- The ward doctors would update the proforma on a daily basis

Measures

Following each out-of-hours shift, the Foundation Programme doctor would provide questionnaire feedback on the effectiveness of the proforma. The following measures would be determined:

Outcome measure

- Time taken for the out-of-hours doctor to gain an accurate impression of the patient admission.
- The satisfaction score of the handover process as perceived by the on-call doctor.
- The proportion of jobs carried out without reviewing any medical records about the patient.

Process measure

- Is there a summary proforma for each patient on the ward?
- Is the proforma being updated on a daily basis?

Balancing measure

- The amount of time spent updating the proforma on a daily basis by the ward doctors versus the amount of time saved by the on-call team by using the proforma.

- Baseline measurements would be taken from 20 Foundation Programme doctors.
- Feedback would be received from 20 Foundation Programme doctors for each PDSA cycle.

Do

The proforma was implemented on the Care of the Elderly ward. Qualitative feedback from the ward doctors and the on-call team highlighted key issues with the proforma:

- Ward doctor: 'There should be an empty 'Notes' box on the proforma to allow different specialties to tailor the list accordingly. For example, on the Care of the Elderly ward, it would be necessary to note the Mini Mental State Examination score and the Do Not Attempt CPR status.'
- On-call doctor: 'The proforma is too busy. There are too many boxes.'

Study

Compared with baseline, all measures recorded showed signs of improvement:

- The outcome measures all improved (Table 25.3).
- The proforma was welcomed by the Care of the Elderly ward doctors and was updated on 96% of occasions.
- It would take on average 7 minutes for the ward doctors to update the list on a daily basis. With an average review of 30 patients during an on-call service, referring to Table 25.3, the proforma saved the on-call doctor approximately 1 hour (30 patients × 2 minutes saved) during his or her 13-hour shift.

Act

With an aim to further improve the outcomes measured, amendments were made to the proforma based on the feedback received from those involved in the project. The PDSA cycle was repeated a further two times, to ensure that all the kinks in making the change work were addressed. The proforma used as part of PDSA cycle 3 is illustrated in Table 25.4. As shown, the layout issues were addressed and a 'Notes' box was added.

Table 25.3 Measurements from Plan-Do-Study-Act (PSDA) Cycle 1.

	Baseline	PDSA Cycle 1
Satisfaction score	2.47	2.95
Time taken to gain accurate impression of patient admission (minutes)	13	11
Jobs carried out without reviewing any medical records (%)	68	32

Table 25.4 Revised proforma – Plan-Do-Study-Act-Cycle 3.

Bed	Demographic information	Presenting complaint and diagnosis	Comorbidities	Operations/ procedures	Current issues:	Management plan	Discharge plan and social issues	Key blood results:	Notes:	Jobs:
1	Rina Kaura 08/02/1922 90 **1111111 111** Admitted: 12/02/12	Shortness of breath LRTI Atrial flutter →T2RF→ BiPAP	1) T2DM-drug 2) MI-09/11 3) AF-on warfarin 4) HTN 5) Hypothyroid	Echo - mild LV impairment LVH Δ cor pulmonale X-ray Rt Shoulder: loss of rotator cuff tendon, degenerative changes	1) Peripheral oedema 2) Pain/ ↓ROM right shoulder 3) Reduced mobility 4) LRTI	Physiotherapy OT Fluid management on co-trimoxazole until 19/02/12	Lives alone, Carer's BD	ANA +'ve (28/02/12) CRP 52 (27/02/12)	MMSE: - AMT 6/6 **DNACPR** TTA: No	
2										

AF, atrial fibrillation; AMT, abbreviated mental test; ANA, anti-nuclear antibody; BD, twice-daily; BiPAP, Bilevel Positive Airway Pressure; CRP, C-reactive protein; DNACPR, do no attempt cardiopulmonary resuscitation; Echo, echocardiography; HTN, hypertension; LRTI, lower respiratory tract infection; LV, left ventricular; LVH, left ventricular hypertrophy; MI, myocardial infarction; MMSE, mini-mental state examination; OT, occupational therapy; ROM, range of motion; T2DM, type 2 diabetes mellitus; T2RF, type 2 respiratory failure; TTA, to take away.

The feedback received as part of each PDSA cycle is graphically displayed in Fig. 25.3. By the end of PDSA cycle 3, all objectives set at the start of the project were successfully accomplished. While the on-call doctor would still need to review the medical records, having the proforma as an adjunct saved the on-call doctor approximately 3.5 hours (30 patients × 7 minutes saved) during his or her 13-hour shift. Having demonstrated the effectiveness of the proforma on a small scale, the next step would be to implement this proforma on other medical and surgical wards.

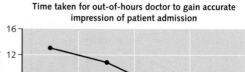

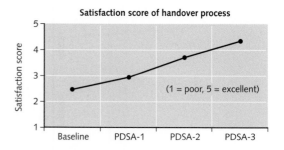

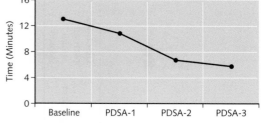

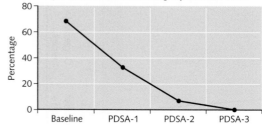

Fig. 25.3 Repeating the Plan-Do-Study-Act (PDSA) cycle.

Chapter Summary

- The first step of a quality improvement project is to decide which area of healthcare you are trying to improve.
- An 'aim' statement should be developed, being specific about the degree of improvement you are expecting to achieve, by when you wish to accomplish this improvement and who (or what system) will be affected.
- To assist organizations in developing an aim statement in a complex clinical setting, the Institute of Medicine put forth six dimensions for improvement in healthcare. Healthcare delivered should be safe, effective, patient centred, timely, efficient and equitable.
- The three main types of measures used in quality improvement are outcome measures, process measures and balancing measures.
- Outcome measures inform us whether the change made has led to an improvement in the outcome we are ultimately trying to improve.
- Process measures the specific steps in a process that lead to a particular outcome.
- Balancing measures inform us whether changes in one part/step of the system are causing 'new' problems in other parts of the system.

- It is useful to draw a flowchart of the steps involved in the current process. This will help you identify any flaws in the system that aren't functioning as planned.
- The Plan-Do-Study-Act (PDSA) cycle approach allows you to test any changes made to the healthcare system using a systematic approach.
- The PDSA cycle involves developing a plan to test the change (Plan), implementing the change (Do), collecting and analysing data to learn from the consequences of the change (Study) and determining what modifications should be made to the current change for the next cycle (Act).

FURTHER READING

Botwinick, L., Bisognano, M., Haraden, C., 2006. Leadership Guide to Patient Safety. IHI Innovation Series white paper. Institute for Healthcare Improvement, Cambridge, MA.

Institute for Healthcare Improvement. How to improve. Available from: http://www.ihi.org/resources/Pages/HowtoImprove/default.aspx [Accessed 21st Septmeber 2018].

Institute of Medicine, 2000. To Err is Human: Building a Safer Health System. National Academy Press, Washington, DC.

Leis, J.A., Shojania, K.G., 2017. A primer on PDSA: executing plan-do-study-act cycles in practice, not just in name. BMJ Qual. Saf. 26 (7), 572–577.

TEACHING THEORY AND PRACTICE

Chapter 26

Medical education 247

Chapter 27

Designing a teaching session and teaching
programme. 253

Chapter 28

Teaching methods 259

Chapter 29

Teaching materials 267

Chapter 30

Evaluation, assessment and feedback 271

Chapter 31

Dealing with the student in difficulty 279

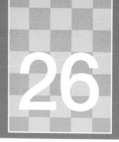
INTRODUCTION

According to the Institute for International Medical Education (IIME), 'medical education is the process of teaching, learning and training of students with an ongoing integration of knowledge, experience, skills, qualities, responsibilities and values which qualify an individual to practice medicine'. Once qualified and registered in a field of practice, most countries require doctors to subsequently provide evidence of continuing professional development (CPD) or continuing medical education throughout their career. The main purpose of CPD is to ensure that doctors provide safe medical practice by keeping up to date with the latest medical research and evidence. Engagement in CPD activities typically involves participating in accredited training courses that are assigned 'credits'. The number of credits offered for a course is broadly related to the duration of the course. Evidence of engagement in CPD activities is also required for revalidation, which is typically undertaken on a 3- to 5-year cycle.

LEARNING PERSPECTIVES/ THEORIES

With a focus on lifelong learning, it is important we understand, both as learners and teachers, how knowledge is absorbed, processed and retained. This requires having a working knowledge and understanding of some of the key learning orientations/theories, including:

1. Behaviourist
2. Cognitivist
3. Humanist
4. Social learning
5. Constructivist

These five learning theories, based on work from Merriam and Caffarella, will be discussed in turn, with examples of how each theory can be applied to medical education practice from a teacher's perspective.

HINTS AND TIPS

We need to understand what our own personal learning theory is in order to understand our own limitations. As a teacher, you should seek to understand the foundation of beliefs of your students to help you adapt your teaching style and actions to maximize student learning.

Behaviourist orientation

This learning orientation is useful:

- for demonstrating technical or psychomotor skills
- for developing competencies
- when a change in behaviour is the desired outcome of a teaching session.

Learning theory

The behaviourist orientation involves a teacher-centred approach to teaching. The three main assumptions central to the learning process are:

- observable behaviour
- manipulating the environment to shape behaviour
- step-wise progression to reinforce transfer of knowledge and skills to the learner.

Translating theory to practice

A behaviourist learning approach is advocated when:

- developing learning objectives:
  - Behavioural learning objectives allow learners to know what behaviour (or performance) will be learned, the conditions necessary for the performance and the evaluation criteria to demonstrate acceptable performance (outlined in Chapter 30).
- designing competency-based curricula:
  - By developing behaviour-orientated learning objectives, the level of competency expected for an element of the curriculum can be determined.

Within medical education, a behaviourist approach is commonly used during the following activities:

- The development and evaluation of clinical skills:
  - The teacher demonstrates a specific desired behaviour or skill (e.g., demonstrates how to perform a cardiovascular examination), the learner observes the manner or technique demonstrated by the teacher, and an evaluation tool (e.g., scoring criteria – please refer to Chapter 30) is used to evaluate the performance of the learner demonstrating the same skill and provide reinforcement.
- Simulated case scenarios (or role plays):
  - The teacher arranges role-play scenarios using standardized patients (or actors) to provide the students an opportunity to practice and perform different skills and techniques under controlled

circumstances. For example, a role play on breaking bad news to an actor with a new diagnosis of cancer.

Cognitivist orientation

The focus of learning is through cognitive structures. To facilitate learning, the learner uses cognitive tools, including insight, memory and perception, to assign meanings to events.

Learning theory

The cognitivist orientation involves the student creating meaningful learning based on his or her thought process rather than on the external environment, the latter being more consistent with a behaviourist orientation approach. The role of the teacher is to:

- facilitate cognitive processing by helping the student learn how to learn
- develop the learner's capacity and skills for effective self-directed learning.

The student acquires learning skills that are relevant in all teaching sessions regardless of the context or topic. The philosophy behind the cognitivist learning orientation is that learning occurs from relating new knowledge to what is already known. This advocates using learning strategies that link different concepts together so that the learner appreciates the structure of knowledge. The process of linking new knowledge to existing knowledge requires critical thinking through reflection.

Translating theory to practice

A cognitivist learning approach is advocated when:

- constructing concept maps:
  - Concept maps are graphics for representing the relationship between multiple different concepts and ideas.
  - Fig. 26.1 illustrates an example of a concept map published in *The American Journal of Medicine*.
  - The process of creating a concept map involves identifying and drawing relationships or connections (with or without linking words) between key issues and concepts.
- developing reflective thinking:
  - Reflection may occur during (reflection 'in' action) or after (reflection 'on' action) a particular experience (or action).
  - Reflection 'for' action refers to reflecting on what has been learned for the future.

Within medical education, a cognitivist approach is commonly used during the following activities:

- Using concept maps to:
  - recall ideas about a particular topic in order to depict complex relationships
  - brainstorm ideas with other learners

- extract core concepts and meanings from various sources of information, including journal articles, text books and ward teaching
- plan the contents of a paper or presentation.
- Reflective thinking can be used in the following environments:
  - lecture halls
  - hospital wards
  - simulation sessions
  - small group sessions.

Within each of these environments, reflection 'in' action, reflection 'on' action and refection 'for' action can all take place. For example, in the hospital setting:

- Reflection 'in' action: evaluating or reflecting on your colleagues' performance whilst you watch them examine a patient.
- Reflection 'on' action: evaluating or reflecting on your own performance after you have examined a patient.
- Reflection 'for' action: using personal reflection (reflection 'on' action) and feedback from others (refection 'in' action) to reflect on how to improve your examination skills.

Humanist orientation

Humanist learning is viewed as a personal act necessary for students to become autonomous and self-directed learners.

Learning theory

The main aim of humanist learning is to address the basic needs of the student in order to work towards them achieving the ultimate need for self-actualization. The motivation is for the student to become an autonomous learner and achieve their full potential. During the process of self-directed learning, the student plans, carries out and then evaluates their own learning experiences. The role of the teacher is to facilitate the development of the student.

Translating theory to practice

In the 1950s, psychologist Abraham Maslow created the Maslow's Hierarchy of Needs where he explained that certain 'lower level' needs must be met before a person is able to satisfy 'higher level' needs (Fig. 26.2).

- Physiological needs
  - At the first level of the hierarchy of evidence, the physiological needs of the students are of utmost importance.
  - This includes meeting basic needs such as food, water and shelter.
  - If physiological needs are not met, the student may not be able to focus fully on learning.
  - As a teacher, you must ensure there is adequate lighting, ventilation, space and refreshments. If the teaching session is going to be relatively long, timetabling in a scheduled toilet break would be wise.

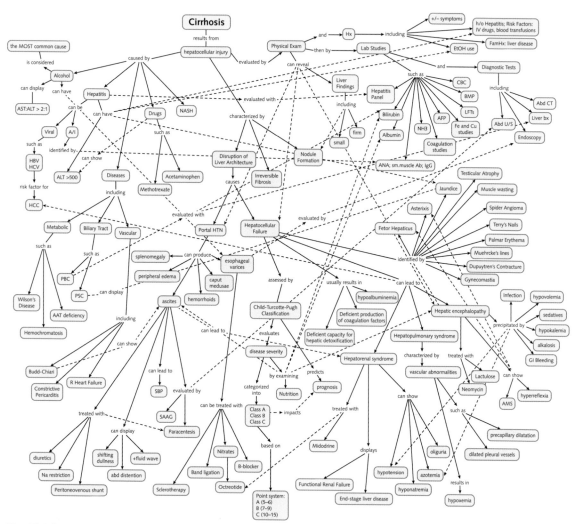

Fig. 26.1 Concept map of cirrhosis. (Reproduced with permission from Torre DM, Daley BJ, Sebastian JL, Elnicki DM. Overview of current learning theories for medical educators. *Am J Med* 2006;119(10):903-907.) *AAT*, alpha-1 antitrypsin; *Abd CT*, abdominal computerised tomography scan; *AFP*, alpha-fetoprotein; *A/I*, auto immune; *ALT*, alanine aminotransferase; *AMS*, altered mental status; *ANA*, antinuclear antibody; *AST*, aspartate aminotransferase; *B-blocker*, Beta-blocker; *BMP*, basic metabolic panel; *bx*, biopsy; *CBC*, complete blood count; *Cu*, copper; *EtOH*, ethanol; *FamHx*, family history; *Fe*, iron; *GI*, gastrointestinal; *HBV*, hepatitis B virus; *HCC*, hepatocellular carcinoma; *HCV*, hepatitis C virus; *h/o*, history of; *HTN*, hypertension; *Hx*, history; *IgG*, immunoglobulin G; *IV*, intravenous; *LFTs*, liver function tests; *Na*, sodium; *NASH*, non-alcoholic steatohepatitis; *NH3*, ammonia; *PBC*, primary biliary cirrhosis; *PSC*, primary sclerosing cholangitis; *R Heart Failure*, Right Heart Failure; *SAAG*, serum ascites albumin gradient; *SBP*, spontaneous bacterial peritonitis; *sm muscle Ab*, smooth muscle antibody; *U/S*, ultrasound.

- Safety needs
  - The students must not only feel physically safe at the teaching venue, but also emotionally and psychologically safe as well.
  - The students should feel free to ask questions and share their ideas without being mocked by their peers or reprimanded by the teacher.
  - As a teacher, remembering the names of your students and involving them in setting ground rules may build mutual trust. Any feedback provided on performance should be done 'constructively'.
- Belonging needs
  - All students must feel:
    - a sense of belonging amongst their peers
    - that they fit in
    - that they are important as an individual and part of the group.

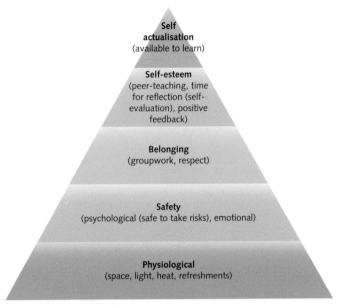

Fig. 26.2 Maslow's hierarchy of needs.

- As a teacher, you can motivate learners:
  - through inclusion and consultation. This is especially important during clinical placements when students frequently feel ignored
  - by seeking, valuing and acting on their input towards the objectives and structure of their teaching sessions
  - by using inclusive learning techniques such as group work.
- Self-esteem needs
  - Several of the points from the previous needs feed directly into the need for self-esteem (or self-confidence) through making the student feel valued.
  - The student is most receptive to learning at this level of the hierarchy, taking responsibility of their own learning.
  - As a teacher, you should get the students involved in learner-centred activities such as peer teaching and peer assessment.
  - Praise and words of appreciation are also important; many positive moments can build self-esteem; however, one unkind comment can destroy it.
- Self-actualization
  - By accounting for all of the other factors at each level of Maslow's hierarchy, the students proactively try to identify ways to fulfil their learning potential, striving for higher learning goals and seeking to achieve them.

HINTS AND TIPS

As a teacher, if you are asked to organize a one-off teaching session with a fresh group of students who you have never taught before, you should attempt to determine what the students know, want to know and expect to learn. Ideally, this should be determined before the start of the teaching session; however, if the teaching is ad-hoc, which is sometimes the case in the clinical setting, you should find out at the start of the teaching session. This demonstrates respect for the learners, which encourages them to engage and participate in the teaching session.

- The higher up in the hierarchy the student is, the better their motivation and therefore the more effective their learning.

Social learning orientation

The key characteristics of the social learning orientation include observation and modelling. Learners assimilate new knowledge through taking on new roles that require role modelling (or mentoring) and practice.

Learning theory

Learners are required to imitate observed behaviours through rehearsal. In comparison to a strict behaviourist approach, social learning theory integrates a cognitive component (further discussed in the 'translating theory to practice' section below). Learners store an image of an observed behaviour in their brain and retrieve that image when they are required to demonstrate the same behaviour. Learning therefore takes place through the interaction between the student, the learning environment and the desired behaviour.

Translating theory to practice

The role of the teacher involves modelling or demonstrating new behaviours and providing students with opportunities to practice these behaviours. The process of role modelling incorporates many of the characteristics of the 'behaviourist' learning orientation. Similar to the example mentioned in the behaviourist section, learners observe a key behaviour of the teacher (e.g., the teacher demonstrates how to perform a cardiovascular examination) and then use these observations to create a memorable model of the behaviour (e.g., the learner remembers exactly what the teacher did and how she or he did it). The next step is for the learner to reproduce the desired behaviour and receive feedback on his or her performance. The unique aspect of the social learning orientation is that role-modelling behaviour is combined with cognitive learning to deepen the student's understanding of the behaviour (e.g., the learner needs to understand not only how to perform a cardiovascular exam, but also why he or she is performing it and what signs they intend to find). Role modelling has been the backbone of teaching practice in clinical medicine for medical students and practicing doctors.

Constructivist orientation

The constructivist learning theory is a relatively new approach to teaching. It involves learning by creating meaning from experiences and assigning significance to them.

Learning theory

The learners critically reflect on their own assumptions, which are based on their own experiences. The teacher assists learners in understanding how to develop their assumptions and assess their validity. The teacher is viewed not as a transmitter of knowledge, but as a guide who facilitates learning.

Translating theory to practice

As student learning is based on prior knowledge, as a teacher you should expose them to new learning experiences in order for them to identify inconsistencies between the students' current understanding and their new experience. Students should be engaged in their learning in an active way, using relevant problems and group interaction. One activity involves:

- Step 1: The student describes a clinical case
- Step 2: The student notes down their thoughts and feelings of the case
- Step 3: At a later date, the student reflects on what they have learned
- Step 4: A small group of students should then come together to discuss similarities and differences in their clinical cases. This step ensures the students test the validity of their assumptions.

Problem-based learning is a constructivist approach to learning (discussed in Chapter 28).

HINTS AND TIPS

The primary aim of constructivism is for learners to 'construct' their own knowledge based on their own experiences. Learning is therefore active rather than passive. The learners make judgements about when and how to modify their knowledge.

OPTIMIZING LEARNING

As a teacher, you should be familiar with the different learning theories in order to create appropriate learning environments to optimize student learning. Table 26.1 provides a summary of when to use each learning style according to the aim of the teaching session.

Table 26.1 How to choose the most effective learning orientation.

General aim of teaching session	Teaching orientation
Performing a new skill	Behavioural
Develop critical thinking and clinical problem-solving skills	Cognitivist
Learners to take responsibility for their own professional development	Humanist (with a focus on self-directed learning)
Learners to demonstrate best practice in the clinical setting	Social learning (learners model expert behaviour)
Problem-based learning involving: - clinical laboratory data - paper-based clinical scenarios - a scientific journal article	Constructivist

HINTS AND TIPS

As a teacher, learning theories form a guide for planning a teaching session. By knowing the general principles of these theories, you are able to use your knowledge more effectively according to the learning activity. For example, if you are planning on demonstrating to students how to perform a clinical examination on a patient, you must decide whether to adopt a behavioural approach (where you demonstrate the examination alone) or a social learning approach (where you demonstrate the examination and also explain what particular signs they need to look out for). What approach you adopt will depend on the experience of the learner and their prior knowledge. As we will discuss in the following chapter, you must always establish the skills and knowledge that the students already possess in order to tailor the level of teaching provided.

● Chapter Summary

- There are three distinct stages in medical education and training: undergraduate education, postgraduate education and continuing professional development.
- With a focus on lifelong learning, it is important we understand, both as learners and teachers, how knowledge is absorbed, processed and retained.
- This requires having a working knowledge and understanding of some of the key learning orientations/theories (behaviourist, cognitivist, humanist, social learning and constructivist).
- The behaviourist orientation involves a teacher-centred approach to teaching.
- The cognitivist orientation involves the student creating meaningful learning based on his or her thought process rather than on the external environment.
- The humanist orientation involves addressing the basic needs of the student in order to work towards them achieving the ultimate need for self-actualization.
- The social learning orientation involves a combination of modelling behaviour and cognitive learning to deepen the student's understanding of the behaviour.
- The constructivist approach involves learning by creating meaning from experiences and assigning significance to them.

FURTHER READING

Kaufman, D.M., 2010. Applying educational theory in practice. In: Cantillon, P., Wood, D. (Eds.), ABC of learning and teaching in medicine, second ed. Blackwell Publishing, Chichester, pp. 1–5.

Kaufman, D.M., 2003. Applying educational theory in practice: ABC of learning and teaching in medicine. BMJ 326, 213–216.

Merriam, S.B., Caffarella, R.S., Baumgartner, L.M., 2006. Learning in adulthood: A comprehensive guide, third ed. Jossey Bass, San Francisco.

Taylor, D.C.M., Hamdy, H., 2013. Adult learning theories: Implications for learning and teaching in medical education: AMEE Guide No. 83. Med. Teach. 35, e1561–e1572.

Torre, D.M., Daley, B.J., Sebastian, J.L., Elnicki, D.M., 2009. Overview of current learning theories for medical eudcators. Adv. Health Sci. Educ. Theory Pract. 14 (5), 791–812.

- level of teaching pitched either too low or high
- humiliating students
- patients not being properly consented
- little opportunity provided for reflection.

As highlighted in Chapter 27, the teacher should ideally plan the teaching session in advance to provide structure and context for the teacher and student. Effective clinical teachers should possess knowledge about:

- the learners
- the subject area
- the patient case scenario used for teaching and knowledge
- how to deliver good-quality teaching using a range of teaching activities based on different learning theories (covered in Chapter 26).

Ward teaching

Teaching on the patient ward round may take place during either 'special teaching' rounds, which are more interactive, or during 'business' rounds, where learning will take place through observation. As most clinical teaching by practicing doctors takes place in the context of a busy clinical workload, a number of steps can be taken to ensure 'effective' time-limited teaching is delivered:

- Step 1: Identify the learner needs by either asking the students or conducting a 2- to 3-minute observation of the learner to help identify learning objectives.
- Step 2: A model for time-limited teaching should be identified. Four examples include:
  - i) The students ask questions based on their specific observations, which are used for discussion
  - ii) The teacher asks a couple of questions based on a student presentation of a previous clinical encounter (e.g., history taking, clinical examination):
    - What do you think might be going on with the patient?
    - What led you to your conclusion?
    Based on the answers received, as a teacher, you need to:
    - reinforce what was done well
    - help the learner identify any errors or omissions
    - focus on teaching a certain aspect of the clinical encounter based on the errors or omissions made (this may involve a follow-up visit to the bedside for further discussion).
  - iii) Observe the student perform a clinical encounter such as history taking, clinical examination or performing a procedural skill.
- Step 3: Provide constructive feedback and highlight areas for future development. Self-evaluation should be encouraged.

COMMON PITFALLS

Key issues commonly encountered with ward teaching include:

- Selecting appropriate patients (those who are not too unwell (or unstable) or those intending to have specific investigations or treatment at the same time as the teaching session)
- Ensuring that the ward staff (sister in charge, ward receptionist, nurses, and so on) know that the teaching session is taking place
- Using a side room for further discussion about a patient rather than bedside or in the ward corridor (which may raise patient confidentiality issues)

Clinic teaching

Learning is limited if students just sit in on a clinic and remain passive observers. Active involvement may include the following:

i) Whilst observing the clinic, the student writes down their observations and thoughts on the clinical encounter; for example, differential diagnosis, investigation approach, management strategy or any questions raised. Any learning points from the patient encounter can be discussed inbetween patients, as well as answering any questions raised by the student.

ii) The student performs the whole or part of the consultation with the teacher listening. The teacher then covers any points with the patient that were not raised by the student. Discussion and feedback between the teacher and student can take place during or after the patient consultation.

iii) The student consults the patient alone, and is subsequently joined by the teacher. The student presents their findings to the teacher (usually with the patient listening, to confirm accuracy), which generates discussion about the patient management plan.

TEACHING LARGE GROUPS/ LECTURING

Whilst we commonly associate 'lecturing' with talking to a large audience, it actually refers to the approach taken to teach rather than the actual number of students being lectured to. Though not common, it is still possible to lecture only five students during a tutorial. Lecturing represents a 'traditional' teaching approach in which the teacher does the majority of the talking. Lectures are regarded as being an efficient teaching method, employing relatively few staff to teach large chunks of the curriculum to a large group of students. Whilst efficient, there is evidence to show that learners attending lectures only retain approximately 5% to 10% of what they hear.

Advantages of large-group teaching/ lecturing

Lectures can reach a big audience quickly

- Lectures can be used to:
  - provide a grounding in a 'new' subject
  - demonstrate how information in a particular area is structured
  - discuss the evidence base behind the topic being covered
  - stimulate curiosity and direct further study.

Disadvantages of large-group teaching

- The communication is mostly one way (from teacher to student)
- It is difficult to give everyone in the group what they expect from the lecture
- The structure of a lecture is usually fairly rigid with limited allowance for interaction or questions
- It is difficult for the teacher to gauge the level of understanding of the students.

Active learning

Active learning in a lecture setting involves the teacher ensuring that steps are taken to facilitate learning rather than just transmitting information (passive learning). An attitude towards active learning in a lecture is therefore promoted, with the teacher encouraging the learner to become more aware of what he or she already knows and to expand their knowledge through thinking and engagement in the material. Various steps can be taken to try and promote active learning during a lecture:

- lecture content
- handouts
- lecture activities.

Lecture content

During the planning phase of the lecture, the teacher should access the students' curriculum and ensure that the material being covered is relevant and fills a gap in the students' knowledge. The principles and concepts of the topic of the lecture should be covered, with analogies and examples, as these are essential for problem solving in the future. Students can be left feeling overwhelmed if a lot of material is covered during a single lecture (less is more). As a teacher, it is important to trust that the learners will add to the minimal core knowledge covered during the lecture through further teaching in small group sessions or during private study.

Handouts

While the standard approach to lecture handouts is to print out the PowerPoint slides (four or six to a page), this is not an effective tool to stimulate learning. If the handout provides all the information contained in the lecture, the students are unlikely to pay attention. Handouts should therefore provide the skeleton of a topic on which the students can build their knowledge on. The handout should be a brief summary of what was contained within the lecture, with partially completed figures and contain questions for further independent study. The lecture handout should encourage the students to listen to the teacher rather than make them spend most the time frantically writing notes. A recommendations list for further reading should be provided.

Lecture activities

The teacher can use a number of activities to keep the students engaged throughout the lecture:

- The students can complete a short quiz at the start of the lecture so that they can assess their own knowledge of the topic. The same (or another) quiz can then be completed near the end of the lecture to hopefully demonstrate learning. Another approach is to mark the quiz, which was completed at the start of the lecture, during the lecture, as relevant topics are discussed.
- Providing summaries of the key points covered, at regular intervals throughout the lecture, can provide an opportunity for learners to reinforce their knowledge or catch up on any material they have missed due to temporary inattention; for example, when they are writing down notes.
- Using multimedia, such as videos, to illustrate a principal or concept, can help to break up the lecture and reengage those students who have disengaged.
- Audience response (or voting) systems are hand-held devices (or clickers) that allow students to indicate their responses to questions posed by the teacher. The results will then appear on the screen as a graph, demonstrating the distribution of all the responses registered.
- Buzz groups involve the teacher asking the students to work in groups of two to four (closet neighbours), for a few minutes, to solve a problem or challenging question set by the teacher. To try and ensure the discussions are all relevant, the teacher should indicate at the start

of the task that a couple of the groups will be asked to feedback to the entire group at the end of the task.

• Brainstorming encourages the students to think about a topic and share their ideas before the teacher shares his or her perspective. After setting a question, all responses from the students are written by the teacher on a whiteboard, blackboard or flip chart. The

teacher can then organize the ideas noted into relevant categories.

• The teacher should ask questions of the class and encourage the students to also ask questions. When the teacher asks the question, it is important to allow enough time for a response (usually 10 seconds), before prompting the audience or selecting a volunteer.

● Chapter Summary

- Small-group, collaborative learning facilitates not only the acquisition of knowledge but also several other skills, such as communication, team-working and problem-solving skills.
- Types of collaborative small-group teaching work include discussion groups, problem-based learning (PBL), case-based learning and simulation.
- Discussion groups allow learners to participate by talking to each other and the teacher during the teaching session. A teacher must think carefully about how he or she plans to 'effectively' facilitate group discussions.
- In PBL, the students use 'triggers' from a problem case scenario to define their own learning objectives. They then conduct independent study before reconvening to discuss and refine their knowledge.
- Case-based learning is an adaption of PBL, whereby written case studies, either prepared by the teacher or brought in by the students, are used to develop clinical reasoning.
- In general terms, simulation is a device or technique that attempts to create characteristics of the real world.
- As most clinical teaching by practicing doctors takes place in the context of a busy clinical workload, a number of steps can be taken to ensure 'effective' time-limited teaching is delivered.
- Lecturing represents a 'traditional' teaching approach in which the teacher does the majority of the talking. Lectures are best used for stimulating interest in a subject and to help direct further learning. Lecture handouts should provide the skeleton of a topic on which the students can build their knowledge on.

FURTHER READING

Brown, G., Manogue, M., 2001. AMEE Medical Education Guide No. 22: refreshing lecturing: a guide for lecturers. Med. Teach. 23, 231–244.

Cleland, J.A., Abe, K., Rethans, J., 2009. The use of simulated patients in medical education. AMEE Guide No. 42. Med. Teach. 31, 477–486.

Dennick, R., Spencer, J., 2011. Teaching and learning in small groups. In: Dornan, T., Mann, K.V., Scherpbier, A.J., Spencer, J. (Eds.), Medical Education Theory and Practice. Churchill Livingstone/Elsevier, Edinburgh, pp. 131–156.

Hargreaves, D.H., Southworth, G.W., Stanley, P., Ward, S.J., 1997. On-the-job Learning for Physicians. Royal Society of Medicine, London.

Irby, D., Wilkerson, L., 2008. Teaching when time is limited. BMJ 336, 384–387.

Long, A., Lock, B., 2014. Lectures and large groups. In: Swanwick, T. (Ed.), Understanding Medical Education: Evidence, Theory and Practice, second ed. ASME/Wiley Blackwell, Chichester, pp. 127–148.

McCrorie, P., 2014. Teaching and learning in small groups. In: Swanwick, T. (Ed.), Understanding Medical Education: Evidence, theory and practice, second ed. Wiley and the Association of Medical Education, Chichester, pp. 123–136.

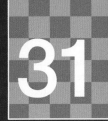
It is inevitable that many of us will struggle or even fail at an activity associated with learning during medical school or during our working life. It is important to recognize this as a normal part of learning. If you never struggle, you are not challenging yourself! If you never make a mistake, you are not learning! Learning from these difficulties and mistakes will allow you to develop your skills in being able to handle further challenges in the future.

Students at university and doctors in clinical practice will have a range of abilities and levels of maturity, as well as different learning techniques. As a teacher, one of your professional roles is to identify and support learners in difficulty. This involves:

- recognizing when a student is in difficulty
- arranging a meeting to investigate the issues behind this difficulty
- suggesting interventions to overcome this difficulty
- assessing the response to your proposed intervention and arranging follow-up.

Each of these steps will now be discussed in turn.

RECOGNITION

There are a number of ways in which students in difficulty may present:

- poor attendance to compulsory and/or noncompulsory teaching sessions
- poor preparation for teaching sessions
- nonengagement in teaching sessions; for example, failure to review or present patients in the clinical setting
- late or absent homework/assessment submission
- frequent written and/or practical examination failure
- unprofessional behaviour; for example, plagiarism, poor attitude towards learning or blaming others.

HINTS AND TIPS

Struggling students may sometimes present in less obvious ways, such as them segregating themselves from a group of fellow students or colleagues, or being reluctant to contribute towards discussions in a teaching session. Other educators who deliver teaching to the same cohort of students may also share similar concerns about a particular student.

WHY DO STUDENTS STRUGGLE ?

Students may present with at least one of the following issues:

- mental illness; for example, anxiety, depression, eating disorders
- personal circumstances; for example, accommodation, money or relationship issues
- inability to balance work and play
- poor study skills; for example, note taking or clinical skills
- poor time-management skills
- specific difficulties with learning; for example, dyslexia
- lack of motivation
- poor revision technique
- poor examination technique; for example, anxiety, irrational beliefs regarding multiple-choice questions ("four B's in a row can't be right?").

These issues may interact with each other; for example, depression linked with a lack of motivation.

CONSULTATION

Having identified a student in potential difficulty, it is important to arrange a meeting with the student to explore possible causes behind any issues that they may be currently facing. As these issues may be complex in nature, it is important to take a holistic approach when exploring possible causes of difficulty. The following areas may be explored:

- *Insight*
  Does the student appreciate that they may have a problem affecting their learning/education?
  What does the student feel may be the cause?
- *Personal circumstances*
  Does the student have a personal situation, such as issues with money, relationships, etc.?
  Is the student able to balance their social life with their educational/work life?
- *Motivation*
  Is the student/doctor still motivated to become/be a doctor?
- *Personal skills*
  Is the student finding time management or organization difficult?
- *Learning*
  What approach does the student take to learning knowledge?

Does the student work regularly throughout the week? Are there issues with learning particular clinical skills? Does the student have concerns about their examination technique?

INTERVENTIONS AND FOLLOW-UP

Following your assessment, it is important to help the student explore solutions to overcome their personal issues.

The most successful interventions are usually those that target specific problem areas (Table 31.1). If you are not the student's tutor, to ensure that the student receives the best support possible, it is important to liaise with the tutor or clinical supervisor, explaining to the student the importance of sharing your concerns. It is important to ensure that any interventions made are followed up. This may involve meeting the student again or emailing them to check on their progress. The General Medical Council provides advice on how to raise concerns and support students in difficulty (please refer to 'Further Reading').

Table 31.1 Interventions for specific student problem areas

Problem	Solution
Mental illness	With the student fully involved, it may be useful to write a letter for the student's general practitioner if an undiagnosed condition, such as dyslexia or depression, is suspected
Specific difficulties with learning	
Personal circumstances	The university usually provides welfare and debt advice
Inability to balance work and play	Regular learning should be planned based on a personal timetable to ensure all learning objectives set by the university are met within a specified time frame
Poor time-management skills	
Poor study skills	Following a university lecture, studying in the library or visiting the wards prior to going home may help to reinforce knowledge
Lack of motivation	An upward spiral of positive emotion and coping can be created by teaching the student how to plan their learning. For example, if attending a heart failure clinic, reading up on the latest relevant heart failure guidelines prior to the clinic would be advocated. Positive, rewarding feedback from the teacher may encourage and motivate further studying
Poor revision technique	The university usually provide one-to-one sessions and workshops to provide learning support. If required, arrangements can also be made to be reviewed by an educational psychologist with access to various psychological therapies such as cognitive behavioural therapy for performance anxiety
Poor examination technique	

● **Chapter Summary**

- As a teacher or tutor, it is important to be able to recognize and support a learner in difficulty.
- Students may struggle due to a number of reasons that may be interacting and complex in nature.
- Arranging a meeting with the student to explore possible causes behind any issues that they may be currently facing is a useful tool.
- It is essential to take a holistic and individualized approach when consulting the student.
- Any interventions made should be followed up with a meeting or email correspondence.

FURTHER READING

Afzal, A., Baber, S., Aly, S., 2015. Student underperformance in health professions education: a risk management perspective to help underperforming students. Adv. Health Prof. Educ. 1 (2), 78–81.

Evans, D., Brown, J., 2010. Supporting students in difficulty. In: Cantillon, P., Wood, D. (Eds.), ABC of learning and teaching in medicine, second ed. Blackwell Publishing, Chichester, pp. 78–82.

Ford, M., Masterton, G., Cameron, H., Kristmundsdottir, F., 2008. Supporting struggling medical students. Clinical Teacher 5 (4), 232–238.

General Medical Council. Supporting medical students with mental health conditions. Available from: https://www.gmc-uk.org/education/undergraduate/23289.asp [Accessed 21st September 2018].

SELF-ASSESSMENT

Single best answer (SBA) questions 283

Extended-matching questions (EMQs) 293

SBA answers 301

EMQ answers 309

Single best answer (SBA) questions

Chapter 7 Handling data

1. Which of the following is not an example of a ratio variable?
   - A. Speed (in m/s).
   - B. Weight (in kg).
   - C. Age (in years).
   - D. Height (in cm).
   - E. Pain scale (1–5).

2. Which of the following is not true about the probability density function of the normal distribution?
   - A. Symmetrical about the mean.
   - B. Defined by the variance of the population.
   - C. Defined by the mean of the population.
   - D. Bell shaped.
   - E. Becomes less peaked as the variance decreases.

3. Which of the following is not true about positively skewed distributions?
   - A. The mass of the distribution is concentrated on the left.
   - B. The median of the distribution is lower than the mode.
   - C. There is a long tail to the right.
   - D. The mean of the distribution is greater than the median.
   - E. The F-distribution has a positively skewed distribution.

4. The following data are on the length of stay (in days) following admission for an acute myocardial infarction in a sample of 10 patients:

   6 12 6 2 17 11 6 3 21 5

   Which of the following measures is correct?
   - A. Mean = 9.8 days.
   - B. Mode = 21 days.
   - C. Range = 23 days.
   - D. Standard deviation = 2.6 days.
   - E. Variance = 38.8 days^2.

Chapter 8 Investigating hypotheses

1. We measure the body weight of a sample of 100 patients admitted to hospital with a myocardial infarction. Below is a table of summary statistics of this sample:

Mean (kg)	Median (kg)	Range (kg)	Standard deviation (kg)
71.4	70.4	60.4–81.4	9.4

   We expect 95% of patients in the population to have a body weight between:
   - A. 50.5 and 70.4 kg.
   - B. 44.5 and 88.5 kg.
   - C. 55.5 and 85.4 kg.
   - D. 53.0 and 89.8 kg.
   - E. 60.4 and 81.4 kg.

2. In a randomized controlled trial investigating the clinical effectiveness of amitopril, a new angiotensin-converting enzyme inhibitor (ACEi), patients with hypertension were randomized to either amitopril or ramipril (the gold standard ACEi). Blood pressure measurements were taken in both treatment groups 1 year following the start of the study. A statistical test comparing blood pressure measurements in both treatment groups showed there was no statistically significant difference between the two groups. The study investigators failed to carry out sample size calculations at the start of the study. It is therefore possible that the study did not have enough power to detect a difference in blood pressure between the two treatment groups (if there truly is a difference to detect). The power refers to the:
   - A. Sample size of the study.
   - B. Probability of a type 2 error.
   - C. Probability of not making a type 1 error.
   - D. Probability of a type 1 error.
   - E. Probability of not making a type 2 error.

3. You want to conduct a study to investigate whether there is a statistically significant relationship between taking drug A and the risk of a myocardial infarction. Which one of the following statements is true regarding the null hypothesis?
   - A. The null hypothesis (H_0) is 'there is a relationship between taking drug A and the risk of a myocardial infarction'.
   - B. Setting the alpha at 0.05, if the statistical analysis for the study shows a $P = 0.03$, the H_0 should not be rejected.
   - C. The H_0 is 'there is no relationship between taking drug A and the risk of a myocardial infarction'.

D. Setting the alpha at 0.05, if the statistical analysis for the study shows a $P = 0.07$, the H_0 should be rejected.
E. The H_0 is the same as the alternative hypothesis in this study.

Chapter 9 Systematic review and meta-analysis

1. The I^2 statistic:
    A. Is commonly used in case–control studies.
    B. Is larger if there is more heterogeneity between studies.
    C. provides an estimate of the proportion of the total variation in effect estimates that is due to homogeneity between studies.
    D. Is based on the z statistic.
    E. Ranges from 0 to 1.

2. The fixed effects meta-analysis:
    A. Is used when there is evidence of statistical heterogeneity between the studies.
    B. Assumes that different studies are estimating different true population exposure effects.
    C. Assumes that there is a single underlying 'true' effect that each study is estimating.
    D. Gives more weight to the smaller studies.
    E. Calculates the weight using the square of the variance of the exposure effect estimate.

3. A research group performed a meta-analysis of case–control and cohort studies investigating whether an association exists between cardiovascular risk factors and venous thromboembolism (VTE). Twenty-one case–control or cohort studies were included, showing the risk of VTE was 1.51 for hypertension, 1.42 for diabetes mellitus and 2.33 for obesity. The group wished to determine whether the findings of the meta-analysis are robust to the methodology used to obtain them. The analysis performed involves omitting low-quality studies. What type of analysis did the research group perform?
    A. Sensitivity analysis.
    B. Statistical heterogeneity analysis.
    C. Subgroup analysis.
    D. Random effects meta-analysis.
    E. Fixed effects meta-analysis.

4. One of the greatest limitations with systematic reviews is that not all studies carried out are published. The main graphical method used for identifying publication bias is by constructing a:
    A. Dot plot.
    B. Funnel plot.
    C. Bar chart.
    D. Histogram.
    E. Forest plot.

5. Which of the following is an agreed method of assessing the quality of reporting systematic reviews and meta-analyses?
    A. National Health Services (NHS).
    B. World Health Organization (WHO).
    C. Preferred Reporting Items for Systematic reviews and Meta-Analyses (PRISMA).
    D. Consolidated Standards of Reporting Trials (CONSORT).
    E. National Institute for Health and Care Excellence (NICE).

Chapter 10 Research design

1. In men with benign prostatic hyperplasia, is laser prostatectomy superior to transurethral resection of the prostate for short-term symptomatic relief? While both treatment options are available to patients, there is currently no evidence that one procedure is more effective than the other. What is the most appropriate research design to investigate this research question?
    A. Case–control study.
    B. Case report.
    C. Cohort study.
    D. Cross-sectional study.
    E. Randomized controlled trial.

2. A research group investigates whether smoking causes a rare blood disorder known as bloodophilia. What is the most appropriate research design to investigate this hypothesis?
    A. Case report.
    B. Cohort study.
    C. Case–control study.
    D. Randomized controlled trial.
    E. Cross-sectional study.

3. Which one of the following types of studies is considered the gold standard to assess the benefits and harms of a therapy?
    A. Case–control study.
    B. Cohort study.
    C. Randomized controlled trial (RCT).
    D. Case report.
    E. Ecological study.

4. Researchers have recently discovered a new neurological disorder that typically presents in healthcare professionals aged over 50 years. However, it is rare, with a prevalence of 1 in 60,000 individuals. Little is known about the aetiology of the disease. It has been postulated to be due to long-term exposure to excessive amounts of caffeine over many years. In order to test this

hypothesis, which of the following study designs would be most useful?

A. Randomized controlled trial (RCT).
B. Prospective cohort study.
C. Case–control study.
D. Case report.
E. Retrospective cohort study.

5. Amitopril, a new angiotensin-converting enzyme inhibitor drug, has recently been licensed, marketed and made available for all patients with hypertension in the UK. The next step is to gather information on whether the drug can be used in combination with other antihypertensive treatments. Which clinical trial phase is warranted?

A. Phase I trial.
B. Phase II trial.
C. Phase III trial.
D. Phase IV trial.
E. Preclinical trial.

6. A doctor hypothesizes that gas emissions from a newly opened factory are causing the recent increase in the number of patients admitted to the local hospital with a respiratory disease. Which of the following factors would most strongly implicate the causal relationship between the gas emissions and respiratory disease?

A. Temporarily closing the factory for 2 months had no impact on the incidence of respiratory disease in the local area.
B. The duration of exposure to the gas emission is related to the risk of respiratory disease.
C. There are no previous studies at other locations to investigate whether a causal relationship exists.
D. No potential biological mechanism has been identified.
E. The incidence of respiratory disease increased before the factory opened.

7. You are interested in investigating whether an association exists between head circumference at birth and IQ at the age of 45 years. What is the most appropriate research design to investigate this research hypothesis?

A. Randomized controlled trial.
B. Case–control study.
C. Retrospective cohort study.
D. Ecological study.
E. Prospective cohort study.

8. To assist with health resource allocation decisions, a research group set out to determine the burden of a particular disease in the population. Which type of study should be undertaken?

A. Randomized controlled trial.
B. Ecological study.

C. Cohort study.
D. Cross-sectional study.
E. Case–control study.

Chapter 11 Randomised controlled trials

1. In randomized controlled trials, the main aim of randomization is to:

A. Reduce cost.
B. Reduce confounding.
C. Reduce bias.
D. Increase the external validity of the results.
E. Reduce the number of patients lost to follow-up.

2. You review the long-term complications of a new antidiabetic treatment for patients with type 2 diabetes mellitus. A study of 5000 patients (2500 treatment, 2500 control) showed that there were 114 patients who had a myocardial infarction in the treatment group and 61 patients who had a myocardial infarction in the control group over the 3-year study period. Which one of the following statements is true?

A. 47 patients would need to be treated for 1 year with the new antidiabetic drug to cause 1 extra myocardial infarction.
B. 53 patients would need to be treated for 3 years with the new antidiabetic drug to prevent 1 extra myocardial infarction.
C. 47 patients would need to be treated for 3 years with the new antidiabetic drug to cause 1 extra myocardial infarction.
D. 53 patients would need to be treated for 1 year with the new antidiabetic drug to cause 1 extra myocardial infarction.
E. 47 patients would need to be treated for 3 years with the new antidiabetic drug to prevent 1 extra myocardial infarction.

3. In a cardiovascular disease prevention trial, patients were randomized to receive either aspirin or a matching placebo and then to either beta-carotene or a different matching placebo. What type of study design has been employed?

A. Crossover trial.
B. Parallel trial.
C. Factorial trial.
D. Cluster trial.
E. Preclinical trial.

4. A recent trial shows that a new asthma treatment reduces the annual rate of admissions for acute exacerbations of asthma by 25% compared with placebo. How many patients will need to be treated to prevent one admission?

A. 50.
B. 4.

C. 5.

D. 40.

E. 6.

Chapter 12 Cohort studies

1. In prospective cohort studies, the biggest drawback is:
   A. Loss to follow-up.
   B. Recruiting enough patients for the study.
   C. Inability to tolerate the intervention.
   D. Confounding.
   E. Expense.

2. Any excess risk of exposure (associated with an occupation) is likely to be underestimated if the unexposed group includes subjects from the general population. The relative risk of the occupational exposure on the disease outcome will therefore be underestimated. This is because, in general:
   A. The general population is healthier than the working population.
   B. The unexposed group is healthier than the exposed group.
   C. The working population is healthier than the general population.
   D. There is no difference between the health of the general population and the working population.
   E. There is no difference between the health of the exposed and unexposed groups.

Chapter 13 Case–control studies

1. A recent case–control study showed that dietary supplementation with omega-3 fatty acids significantly reduced the odds of cardiovascular deaths (odds ratio 0.87, 95% confidence interval 0.79–0.95, $P = 0.002$). An odds ratio of 0.87 means:
   A. Omega-3 fatty acids reduce the odds of cardiovascular deaths by 87%.
   B. Omega-3 fatty acids reduce the odds of cardiovascular deaths by 87 times.
   C. Omega-3 fatty acids reduce the odds of cardiovascular deaths by 13%.
   D. Omega-3 fatty acids reduce the odds of cardiovascular deaths by 13 times.
   E. Omega-3 fatty acids increase the odds of cardiovascular deaths by 87%.

2. In a case–control study, men aged between 50 and 60 years with lung cancer were selected as cases. How many control subjects should be selected to improve the statistical power of the study to detect a difference between cases and controls?
   A. One control should be selected for every case.
   B. Two controls should be selected for every case.
   C. Three controls should be selected for every case.

D. Four controls should be selected for every case.

E. Five controls should be selected for every case.

3. Which of the following statements is not true about the odds ratio and risk ratio?
   A. When the disease is not rare, the odds ratio can underestimate the risk ratio.
   B. Odds and odds ratio are usually calculated in case–control studies.
   C. When the disease is rare, the odds ratio is approximately equal to the risk ratio.
   D. Risk and risk ratio are usually calculated in cohort studies.
   E. In general, the odds ratio is interpreted in the same way as the risk ratio.

4. A case–control study investigates the association between smoking and myocardial infarction (MI). If cases who were smokers die more quickly, there will be a lower frequency of smokers amongst the remaining cases. This will:
   A. Underestimate the association between smoking and myocardial infarction (MI). This will confound the study results.
   B. Have no effect on the association between smoking and MI.
   C. Overestimate the association between smoking and MI. This will bias the study results.
   D. Overestimate the association between smoking and MI. This will confound the study results.
   E. Underestimate the association between smoking and MI. This will bias the study results.

Chapter 14 Measures of disease occurrence and cross-sectional studies

1. A population initially contains 30,000 people free of disease and 1324 people develop diabetes (300 have type 1 diabetes and 1024 people have type 2 diabetes) over 2 years of observation. The incidence risk of type 1 diabetes over the 2-year period was:
   A. 1.7%.
   B. 1.0%.
   C. 4.4%.
   D. 0.05%.
   E. 0.5%.

2. A total of 4000 women attended their local breast cancer screening service and were found to not have breast cancer. Over the following 3 years, 39 of these women were diagnosed with breast cancer. The incidence rate of breast cancer among the 4000 women is:
   A. 975 cases.
   B. 975 cases per 100,000 person-years.
   C. 39 cases per 4000 person-years.

D. 325 cases per 100,000 person-years.
E. 325 cases.

3. A research group distributes a health survey to investigate the prevalence of depression in West London. Only 70% of the study population replied to the survey. Which factor is not associated with a low response rate?
    A. Alcohol or drug misuse.
    B. More unwell.
    C. Male sex.
    D. Younger age.
    E. Higher socioeconomic status.

Chapter 15 Ecological studies

1. The graph underneath shows the mortality rate from stroke according to cholesterol level for four different countries. The scatter for each country displays the association between cholesterol level and stroke mortality rate at an individual level. Regarding the association between cholesterol level and stroke mortality rate, there is:

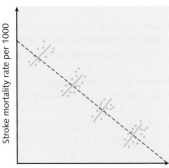

A. No association.
B. No ecological fallacy.
C. Ecological fallacy – negative bias.
D. Ecological fallacy – positive bias.
E. Ecological fallacy – reversal of association.

Chapter 16 Case report and case series

1. Case reports are most useful when:
    A. The sample size of your study is large.
    B. Determining a cause–effect relationship between an intervention and outcome.
    C. Developing new practice guidelines.
    D. Unknown manifestations of a known disease are identified.
    E. The sample size of your study is small.

2. A case series:
    A. Is a descriptive study that reports on data from a group of individuals who have a similar disease.

B. Can be prospective or retrospective and usually involves only a small number of individuals.
C. Can only include consecutive individuals (all cases) with the same disease.
D. A and B only.
E. A, B and C.

Chapter 17 Qualitative research

1. In qualitative research, which of the following refers to reviewing and analysing the data in conjunction with data collection?
    A. Saturation point.
    B. Snowball sampling.
    C. Quota sampling.
    D. Iterative approach.
    E. Triangulation.

2. In a qualitative study of chronic heart failure patients' understanding of their symptoms and drug therapy, all but one participant described how prescribed medications had improved their symptoms. This one patient attributed his symptom improvement to a herbal remedy. When analysing the data, all cases were reviewed. What type of sampling method was used?
    A. Quota sampling.
    B. Negative sampling.
    C. Snowball sampling.
    D. Maximum variation sampling.
    E. Positive sampling.

3. A qualitative study is carried out to investigate the attitudes of medical students on the feedback they receive from their medical school on exam performance. The researchers openly acknowledge (and address) that the relationship among the researchers, the research topic and subjects may have influenced the study results. This concept is known as:
    A. Triangulation.
    B. Iteration.
    C. Grounding.
    D. Reflexivity.
    E. Transferability

Chapter 18 Confounding

1. A randomized controlled trial randomly allocated patients with hypertension to either a new antihypertensive drug or a placebo drug. Two months following the start of the trial, blood pressure measurements were significantly lower in the new treatment group than in the placebo group ($P = 0.023$). However, at the start of the study, the average body mass index (BMI) of patients in the new drug group was lower than the BMI of patients

in the placebo drug group. This difference in BMI between the two groups may have contributed to the statistically significant difference observed in blood pressure measurements. When analysing the study results, which of the following is correct?

A. Body mass index (BMI) is definitely not a confounding factor so the results must be correct.

B. BMI may be a confounding variable and should be corrected for using a stratified analysis approach.

C. All patients in both groups with a BMI greater than 30 (considered as obese) should be excluded from the study analysis.

D. BMI may be a confounding factor so the trial should be repeated, ensuring that recruitment is restricted to those patients with a BMI less than 30.

E. As the trial is randomized, the results must be correct and the differences in BMI between the two treatment groups can be ignored.

2. In a study comparing the drug kavitab to placebo on the risk of myocardial infarction, the crude risk ratio in the drug group was 0.31. The investigators stratify the data according to gender. The stratum-specific risk ratio of myocardial infarction amongst the male and female patients was 0.12 and 0.67, respectively. Which of the following statements is true?

A. There is no association between the drug kavitab and myocardial infarction.

B. Gender is a confounding factor.

C. Kavitab is an effect modifier.

D. Gender is an effect modifier.

E. Kavitab is a confounding factor.

Chapter 19 Screening, diagnosis and prognosis

1. A total of 1234 patients known to have a disease were tested using a new diagnostic test and 567 patients test positive. Furthermore, 1234 patients without the disease were tested and 1145 return a negative result. Which of the following statements is true regarding the outcome of this analysis?

A. The sensitivity of the new diagnostic test is 54.1%.

B. The specificity of the new diagnostic test is 7.2%.

C. The positive predictive value of the new diagnostic test is 13.6%.

D. The negative predictive value of the new diagnostic test is 63.2%.

E. The sensitivity of the new diagnostic test is 41.9%.

2. The most clinically useful measure that helps inform the likelihood of having a disease in a patient with a positive result from a diagnostic test is the:

A. Sensitivity.

B. Confidence interval.

C. Specificity.

D. Positive predictive value.

E. P-value.

3. A new blood test for diagnosing patients with syphilis infection was trialled in a high-prevalence syphilis population. The specificity and sensitivity of the test were found to be 97% and 88%, respectively. The health authorities are thinking about trialling the new test in a population with a low prevalence of syphilis. How will this affect the performance of the diagnostic test?

A. The sensitivity of the test will be lower in the low-prevalence population.

B. The negative predictive value is higher in the low-prevalence population.

C. The specificity of the test will be higher in the low-prevalence population.

D. The positive predictive value is higher in the low-prevalence population.

E. There is no change to the sensitivity, specificity, negative predictive value or positive predictive value.

4. When assessing the validity of a diagnostic study, it is important to consider whether the study design may have been affected by potential biases. Partial verification bias:

A. Occurs when only cases with a limited range of disease spectrum are recruited for the study.

B. Occurs when the decision to perform the reference test on an individual is based on the results of the diagnostic study test.

C. May be avoided if the study test is always performed prior to the reference test.

D. Occurs when different reference tests are used to verify the results of the study test.

E. Can always be prevented if a diagnostic study is carefully designed.

5. A research group wishes to determine the diagnostic accuracy of the two verbally asked questions for screening for depression:

• During the past month, have you often been bothered by feeling down, depressed, or hopeless?

• During the past month, have you often been bothered by little interest or pleasure in doing things?

The group compared the performance of this study test against the International Classification of Disease (ICD) diagnostic criteria (reference test). Using the data in the following table, what is the sensitivity of the two-question screening test for depression?

		ICD depression diagnostic criteria: depression?		
		Yes	No	Total
Two-question screen: depression?	Yes	44	140	184
	No	9	307	316
	Total	53	447	500

A. 17.0%.
B. 100.0%.
C. 75.7%.
D. 83.0%.
E. 91.4%.

6. A research group wishes to determine the diagnostic accuracy of the two verbally asked questions for screening for depression:
   - During the past month, have you often been bothered by feeling down, depressed, or hopeless?
   - During the past month, have you often been bothered by little interest or pleasure in doing things?

   The group compared the performance of this study test against the International Classification of Disease (ICD) diagnostic criteria (reference test). Using the data in the following table, what is the specificity of the two-question screening test for depression?

		ICD depression diagnostic criteria: depression?		
		Yes	No	Total
Two-question screen: depression?	Yes	44	140	184
	No	9	307	316
	Total	53	447	500

A. 68.7%.
B. 91.3%.
C. 84.0%.
D. 15.0%.
E. 76.9%.

7. A research group wishes to determine the diagnostic accuracy of the two verbally asked questions for screening for depression:
   - During the past month, have you often been bothered by feeling down, depressed, or hopeless?
   - During the past month, have you often been bothered by little interest or pleasure in doing things?

   The group compared the performance of this study test against the International Classification of Disease (ICD) diagnostic criteria (reference test). The results are as follow:

		ICD depression diagnostic criteria: depression?		
		Yes	No	Total
Two-question screen: depression?	Yes	44	140	184
	No	9	307	316
	Total	53	447	500

Suppose a 44-year-old woman answers 'yes' to both the screening questions for depression. The prevalence of depression in the population is 10%. Using the data in the table above, what is the probability of her actually having depression?

A. 93.4%.
B. 22.5%.
C. 29.6%.
D. 10.0%.
E. 68.4%.

Chapter 20 Statistical techniques

1. The table below displays a contingency table with the results of a randomized controlled trial investigating the incidence of coronary artery restenosis within 3 months after angioplasty with either a bare metal stent (control group) or drug-eluting stent (intervention group). What is the expected frequency, if there is no difference between the two treatments, for the number of patients randomized to the bare metal stent who get coronary artery restenosis within 3 months after angioplasty?

		Restenosis within 3 months after angioplasty		
		Yes	No	Total
Treatment group	Drug-eluting stent	124	301	425
	Bare metal stent	155	270	425
	Total	279	571	850

A. 155.
B. 139.5.
C. 69.75.
D. 279.
E. 289.

2. Which one of the following statements about study sample size is correct when considering the most appropriate statistical test for your data?
   A. When the sample size of a study is small, parametric tests are robust when analysing data that do not follow a Gaussian distribution.

B. When the sample size of a study is small, normality tests have high power to detect whether a sample comes from a Gaussian distribution.
C. When the sample size of a study is small, nonparametric tests have little power to detect a significant difference.
D. When the sample size is large, nonparametric tests have much less power than parametric tests when analysing data that follow a Gaussian distribution.
E. When dealing with large sample sizes, the decision to choose a parametric or nonparametric test matters more.

3. In a study investigating the clinical effectiveness of amitopril, a new angiotensin-converting enzyme inhibitor drug, blood pressure measurements were taken prior to administering amitopril and repeated in the same subjects one month later. What statistical test should be used to test the hypothesis that amitopril lowers blood pressure?
A. Unpaired t-test.
B. Chi-squared test.
C. Mann–Whitney U test.
D. Fisher exact test.
E. Paired t-test.

4. A large multicentre randomized controlled trial was conducted on patients newly diagnosed with breast cancer to evaluate the effect of a new breast cancer drug on 6-month mortality compared with standard drug treatment. The results of the trial are presented below. What statistical test should be

	Alive at 6 months		
	Yes	No	Total
New drug	412	88	500
Standard drug	354	146	500
Total	766	234	1000

used to compare the outcome between the two treatments?
A. Fisher exact test.
B. Unpaired t-test.
C. Chi-squared test.
D. Quality-adjusted life year analysis.
E. Paired t-test.

Chapter 21 Economic evaluation

1. A research group wishes to determine whether drug A is more cost effective than drug B in treating depression. They gather the following information about each treatment:

Treatment	Cost	Effect (number of weeks patient has no depression)
Drug A	£7000	70 weeks
Drug B	£13,000	80 weeks

What is the cost-effectiveness ratio for drug B?
A. £100/week.
B. £50/week.
C. £325/week.
D. £35/week.
E. £162.50/week.

2. A research group wishes to determine whether drug A is more cost effective than drug B in treating depression. They gather the following information about each treatment:

Treatment	Cost	Effect (number of weeks patient has no depression)
Drug A	£7000	70 weeks
Drug B	£13,000	80 weeks

What is the incremental cost-effectiveness ratio for drug B?
A. £1000 per additional week free of depression.
B. £450 per additional week free of depression.
C. £30 per additional week free of depression.
D. £1200 per additional week free of depression.
E. £600 per additional week free of depression.

3. A research group wishes to determine whether drug A is more cost effective than drug B in treating depression. They gather the following information about each treatment:

Treatment	Cost	Effect (number of weeks patient has no depression)
Drug A	£7000	70 weeks
Drug B	£13 000	80 weeks

The NHS trust decides to finance drug B instead of drug A for first-line drug treatment of depression. The opportunity cost is:

A. The cost (financial and nonfinancial) of providing drug A as a second-line drug treatment for depression.

B. The cost (financial and nonfinancial) of what is lost when drug A is not provided as first-line drug treatment for depression.

C. The cost (only financial) of what is lost when drug A is not provided as first-line drug treatment for depression.

D. The cost (financial and nonfinancial) of providing drug B instead of drug A as first-line drug treatment for depression.

E. The cost (only financial) of providing drug A as a second-line drug treatment for depression.

Chapter 24 Clinical audit

1. In a clinical audit, current clinical practice should be compared to a defined set of explicit criteria. Which of the following descriptions of the explicit criteria is not true?
A. Reflect worst practice.
B. Evidence based.
C. Measurable.
D. Cover the structure of care.
E. Cover the outcome of care.

2. Which of the following is not true about clinical audits?
A. Clinical audit is an ongoing process involving a number of audit cycles evaluating the same clinical standards.
B. The results are compared with standards that define best practice.
C. The results are generalizable.
D. Clinical audits never involve randomly allocating patients to different interventions.
E. The aim of clinical audit is to determine whether current local practice resembles best practice.

Chapter 25 Quality improvement

1. The majority of medical errors in healthcare practice are due to:
A. Doctor errors.
B. Faulty systems and processes.
C. Team errors.
D. Nursing errors.
E. Managerial errors.

2. A foundation doctor carries out a quality-improvement project on access to out-patient appointments. As part of the project, she measures the average daily clinician hours available for appointments. What type of measure is she measuring?
A. Outcome measure.
B. Sample measure.
C. Balancing measure.
D. Process measure.
E. Population measure.

3. A pharmacist carries out a quality-improvement project on the number of adverse drug events on the cardiology ward over the past month. She records that there were 8 drug events per 100 doses. Following a series of tutorials on 'good prescribing practice' for the junior doctors on the ward, the pharmacist checks to see whether this education may have led to a reduction in the number of adverse drug events on the same cardiology ward. What type of measure is the pharmacist measuring?
A. Outcome measure.
B. Sample measure.
C. Balancing measure.
D. Process measure.
E. Practice measure.

4. A medical student at East Hospital carries out a quality-improvement project assessing the average glycated haemoglobin (HbA1c) level in a population of patients with diabetes. Having carried out a number of Plan-Do-Study-Act cycles, there is a gradual improvement in the average HbA1c level compared with baseline. A registrar at West Hospital wishes to implement similar changes at his hospital setting. Which one of the following statements is correct?
A. There will be more resistance by healthcare staff to repeat the project at West Hospital as the changes have been already shown to be effective at East Hospital.
B. The registrar should repeat the quality-improvement project at West Hospital, despite there being evidence that the changes were effective at East Hospital.
C. As the changes were shown to be cost effective at East Hospital, the changes will be cost effective at West Hospital.
D. Considering the changes led to an improvement in the average glycated haemoglobin (HbA1c) level in the population of patients at East Hospital, there will be a similar improvement in the average HbA1c level in the population of patients at West Hospital.
E. When implementing changes 'on a large scale', it is unnecessary to first test the changes out on a smaller scale.

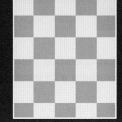

Chapter 7 Handling data

Describing the frequency distribution

A. Median.
B. Range.
C. Arithmetic mean.
D. Reference range.
E. Interquartile range.
F. Standard deviation.
G. Standard error.
H. Geometric mean.
I. Confidence interval.
J. Mode.

For each scenario below, choose the most likely corresponding option from the list given above. Each answer can be used once, more than once or not at all.

1. Adding up all the values in a set of observations and dividing this by the number of values in that set.
2. The middle value when the data are arranged in order of size.
3. A measure of the spread (or scatter) of sample means around the true population mean.
4. The range of values that includes the middle 50% of values when the data are arranged in order of size.
5. A measure of the spread (or scatter) of observations about the mean.

Types of variables

A. Nominal.
B. Distribution.
C. Qualitative.
D. Ratio.
E. Discrete.
F. Multinomial.
G. Ordinal.
H. Frequency.
I. Interval.
J. Dichotomous.

For each of the following examples of variables, select the *best-suited* type of variable it represents from the list of options. Each answer can be used once, more than once or not at all.

1. Gender.
2. Dates.
3. Disease staging.
4. Height.
5. Marital status; i.e., single, married, divorced.

Chapters 8, Investigating hypotheses and 20, Statistical techniques

Extrapolating from sample to population – working with proportions

A. −12.4% to −4.6%.
B. 18.4% to 26.0%.
C. −13.8% to −4.0%.
D. 16.8% to 28.4%.
E. 10.2% to 16.4%.
F. −8.9%.
G. −4.45%.
H. 34.5% to 47.5%.
I. Chi-squared test.
J. Unpaired t-test.

The results of a randomized controlled trial examining the effect of a new cholesterol-lowering drug, statstatin, on the 5-year incidence of myocardial infarction in patients with high cholesterol are as follows:

	Myocardial infarction	No myocardial infarction	Total
Statstatin	60	390	450
Simvastatin	103	362	465
Total	163	752	915

For each question below, choose the most likely corresponding option from the list given above. Each answer can be used once, more than once or not at all.

1. What is the 95% confidence interval of the percentage of cases of myocardial infarction in the statstatin group?
2. What is the 95% confidence interval of the percentage of cases of myocardial infarction in the simvastatin group?
3. What is the difference between the percentage of cases of myocardial infarction in the two treatment groups?
4. What is the 95% confidence interval of the difference in the percentage of cases of myocardial infarction in the two treatment groups?
5. What statistical test should be used to compare the percentage of cases of myocardial infarction in the two treatment groups?

Extrapolating from sample to population – working with means

A. −0.6.
B. 0.0227.
C. 0.0113.
D. 0.0233.
E. 0.5.
F. −0.65 to −0.55.
G. 0.32 to 0.42.
H. One-way ANOVA.
I. Paired *t*-test.
J. Unpaired *t*-test.

A hypothetical randomized controlled trial was set out to examine the effect of a new cholesterol-lowering drug, statstatin, on the incidence of myocardial infarction in patients with high cholesterol. In total, 1000 patients with high cholesterol were randomized to receive either the intervention, statstatin ($n = 500$), or usual treatment for high cholesterol, simvastatin ($n = 500$), with 5-year follow-up data obtained for 450 and 465 patients, respectively. The mean cholesterol level (and standard deviation) 5 years after the start of the study was 3.6 mmol/L (0.24 mmol/L) and 4.2 mmol/L (0.49 mmol/L) in the statstatin and simvastatin groups, respectively. For each question below, choose the most likely corresponding option from the list given above. Each answer can be used once, more than once or not at all.

1. What is the standard error of the mean cholesterol level in the statstatin group?
2. What is the standard error of the mean cholesterol level in the simvastatin group?
3. What is the difference between the mean cholesterol level in the two treatment groups?
4. What is the 95% confidence interval of the difference in mean cholesterol level in the two treatment groups?
5. Assuming the data follow a normal distribution, what statistical test should be used to compare the mean cholesterol level in the two treatment groups?

Chapter 9 Systematic review and meta-analysis

5. Meta-analyses

A. Subgroup analysis.
B. Forest plot.
C. −15, 95% CI −20 to −10.
D. 0, 95% CI −30 to 20.
E. Fixed effects.
F. Funnel plot.
G. Statistical heterogeneity.
H. −25, 95% CI −30 to −20.

I. Random effects.
J. Sensitivity analysis.

A research group performs a meta-analysis of clinical trials investigating the effect of group exercise versus a single workout routine on systolic systemic blood pressure. The figure underneath presents the results of the meta-analysis. Each answer can be used once, more than once or not at all.

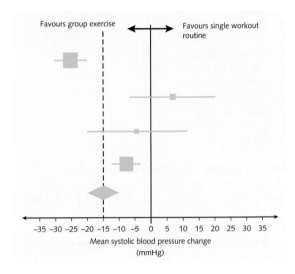

For each question below, choose the most likely corresponding option from the list given above.

1. What is the name of the plot shown in the figure?
2. Considering the I^2 statistic calculated showed no evidence of heterogeneity between the studies, what method was used to calculate the pooled estimate?
3. What is the summary effect estimate of the meta-analysis?
4. What type of plot should the research group construct in order to detect any potential publication bias?
5. The investigators feel that two of the trials included in the meta-analysis are of low quality. What type of analysis should the research group perform to determine whether the meta-analysis findings are robust after excluding these low-quality studies?

Chapter 10 Research design

Study design

A. Systematic review.
B. Randomized controlled trial.
C. Retrospective cohort study.
D. Qualitative study.
E. Ecological study.
F. Case–control study.
G. Prospective cohort study.

H. Meta-analysis.
I. Cross-sectional study.
J. Case series.

For each of the following studies, select the appropriate study design employed from the list given above. Each answer can be used once, more than once or not at all.

1. To determine whether selective serotonin-reuptake inhibitors (SSRIs) are implicated in the aetiology of persistent pulmonary hypertension, infants with the condition were matched with infants without pulmonary hypertension. Rates of past exposure to SSRIs were then recorded.
2. To determine the long-term effectiveness of the influenza vaccine in elderly people, vaccinated and unvaccinated individuals were recruited and followed up over time. Hospitalization rates for pneumonia or influenza were recorded.
3. The effects of raloxifene on fracture risk in postmenopausal women were studied. Subjects were recruited and randomly allocated to either raloxifene or a placebo drug. The study participants were followed up over 5 years and new cases of vertebral fracture recorded in each group.
4. A retrospective review of the evidence for thrombolytic therapy in the prevention of myocardial infarction was carried out. The results from all studies identified were pooled together and a summary estimate calculated.
5. The relationship between an area measure of socioeconomic status and the density of fast food outlets was determined. Different areas across England were compared.

Chapters 10, Research design and 14, Measures of disease occurrence and cross-sectional studies

Measures of disease occurrence

A. Analytical cross-sectional study.
B. Case–control study.
C. 0.025.
D. 19.8%.
E. 0.25.
F. Descriptive cross-sectional study.
G. 9.2%.
H. 80.2%.
I. 0.11.
J. 90.8%.

Patients registered with a number of general practitioners practices were, with their consent, interviewed by telephone to ascertain whether they were depressed and whether they engaged in online social networking. The results are displayed in the table below:

		Depression		
		Yes	No	Total
Social networking profile	Yes	40	394	434
	No	130	32	162
	Total	170	426	596

For each question below, choose the most likely corresponding option from the list given above. Each answer can be used once, more than once or not at all.

1. What study design was used to investigate the burden of depression amongst subjects with and without an online social networking profile?
2. What is the prevalence of depression in subjects who have a social networking profile?
3. What is the prevalence of depression in subjects who don't have a social networking profile?
4. What is the prevalence odds ratio?
5. What is the prevalence ratio?

Chapter 11 Randomized controlled trials

Randomized controlled trials

A. Cluster trial.
B. Blinding.
C. Clinical equipoise.
D. Randomization.
E. Allocation concealment.
F. Selection bias.
G. Measurement bias.
H. Factorial trial.
I. Crossover trial.
J. Superiority trial.

For each scenario below, choose the most likely corresponding option from the list given above. Each answer can be used once, more than once or not at all.

1. The patients and the investigators enrolling the patients cannot foresee treatment group assignment.
2. The patients and investigators (including those involved in recruitment and assessing the outcome) have no knowledge of treatment allocation.
3. Healthcare professionals treating the patients have sufficient doubt about the relative effectiveness of the treatments being compared in the randomized controlled trial.

4. In a trial in which patients were randomized to receive the intervention ($n = 100$) or usual care ($n = 100$), 6 months of follow-up were achieved for 70 and 91 patients, respectively.
5. In a specific type of trial, groups of patients, clinics or communities are randomized to receive the intervention or a control.

Chapters 11, Randomized controlled trials, 12, Cohort studies and 13 Case–control studies

Calculating the strength of an association

A. 0.541.
B. −0.413.
C. 0.133.
D. 13.1.
E. 0.493.
F. 0.154.
G. 0.184.
H. 0.602.
I. 11.2.
J. −0.333.

A hypothetical randomized controlled trial set out to examine the effect of a new cholesterol-lowering drug, statstatin, on the incidence of myocardial infarction in patients with high cholesterol. In total, 1000 patients with high cholesterol were randomized to receive either the intervention, statstatin ($n = 500$) or usual treatment for high cholesterol, simvastatin ($n = 500$), with 5-year follow-up data obtained for 450 and 465 patients, respectively. The primary outcome was the proportion of patients who suffered a myocardial infarction during the follow-up period. Of those who received statstatin, 60 patients had a myocardial infarction compared with 103 patients from the simvastatin group.

For each question below, choose the most likely corresponding option from the list given above. Each answer can be used once, more than once or not at all.

1. What are the odds of having a myocardial infarction in the statstatin group?
2. What is the risk of having a myocardial infarction in the statstatin group?
3. What is the odds ratio of having a myocardial infarction in the statstatin group compared with the simvastatin group?
4. What is the risk ratio of having a myocardial infarction in the statstatin group compared with the simvastatin group?
5. What is the number needed to treat with statstatin instead of simvastatin to prevent one myocardial infarction?

Bias

A. Confounding.
B. Healthy worker effect bias.
C. Berkson's bias.
D. Loss-to-follow-up bias.
E. Recall bias.
F. Random misclassification bias.
G. Follow-up bias.
H. Nonresponse bias.
I. Interviewer bias.
J. Reverse causality.

For each of the following scenarios, select the most appropriate type of bias implicated from the list given above. Each answer can be used once, more than once or not at all.

1. A case–control study to investigate the association between passive smoking and asthma was conducted. Cases (newly diagnosed individuals with asthma) were compared with controls (random sample of individuals without asthma) with regard to exposure to smoke from smokers over the previous 15 years. What type of bias may occur when collecting these data?
2. A case–control study to investigate the association between smoking and diabetes was conducted. Hospitalized patients with diabetes (cases) were compared with hospitalized patients without diabetes (controls). Considering hospitals contain a higher proportion of smokers than the general population, what type of bias may occur?
3. A cohort study to investigate the association between smoking and hair loss was conducted. To measure the exposure status, subjects were classified into groups based on the number of cigarettes smoked per day. What type of bias may occur when collecting this data?
4. A randomized controlled trial to investigate the effect of a new treatment on hypertension was conducted. The investigator is aware of which treatment arm (intervention versus control) participants were randomized to. What type of bias may occur when the investigator takes blood pressure measurements from the study participants?
5. A randomized controlled trial where participants were randomized to medical or surgical therapy for benign prostatic hyperplasia was conducted. If patients undergoing surgical treatment do well (i.e., the symptoms of benign prostatic hypertrophy, such as intermittent micturition, resolve) and do not return for follow-up, what type of bias may be introduced?

Chapters 12, Cohort studies and 18,

Confounding

Confounding

A. 3.0.
B. Sensitivity analysis.
C. Case–control.
D. Stratification.
E. Cohort.
F. Cross-sectional.
G. Hip fracture.
H. Death.
I. 2.01.
J. 0.03.
K. There is a strong association between bedsores and death.
L. There is a weak association between bedsores and death.
M. There is no association between bedsores and death.

A research group carries out a study investigating whether an association exists between the development of new bedsores and death among patients admitted to the orthopaedic ward with neck of femur fractures. All such admissions were included in the study. The study participants were then followed up during their hospital stay to see whether they survived until discharge. The study results are shown in the table underneath

		Death		
		Yes	No	Total
Bed sores	Yes	32	202	234
	No	35	733	768
	Total	67	935	1002

For each question below, choose the most likely corresponding option from the list given above. Each answer can be used once, more than once or not at all.

1. What study design was used to investigate the association between bedsores and death?
2. What is the risk ratio?
3. The research group suspected that those patients with many comorbidities were more likely to acquire bedsores than those with a few or no comorbidities. To be considered as a confounding variable, the comorbidity variable must also be associated with which variable?
4. All patients recruited were categorized into two separate subgroups (medically unwell versus medically well) based on the number/severity of their comorbid conditions. A table similar to that above was

subsequently constructed for each subgroup. What is the name of this type of analysis?
5. The risk ratio for death in the presence of bedsores was 1.02 in the medically unwell subgroup and 1.0 in the medically well subgroup. What conclusion can be reached from the study results?

Chapter 15 Ecological studies

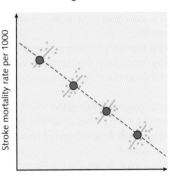

A   Cholesterol level

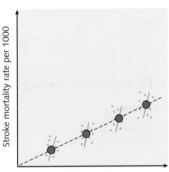

B   Cholesterol level

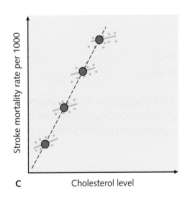

C   Cholesterol level

Ecological studies

A. $r = 0$.
B. $r = -1.0$.
C. $r = 1.0$.
D. $r = 0.7$.
E. Positive bias.
F. Reversal of association.

G. Negative bias.
H. No bias.
I. r = −0.7.
J. r = 1.3.

Scatter plots A to C displays the results of a hypothetical study investigating the relationship between cholesterol level and stroke mortality rate. Each red dot represents group data from a country. The orange dots represent individual patient level data for each respective country.
For each of the following questions, select the most likely corresponding option from the list given above. Each answer can be used once, more than once or not at all.

1. Referring to graph A, what is the Pearson correlation coefficient (r) for the individual patient level data?
2. Referring to graph A, what type of ecological fallacy bias is displayed?
3. Referring to graph B, what is the Pearson correlation coefficient (r) for the individual patient level data?
4. Referring to graph B, what type of ecological fallacy bias is displayed?
5. Referring to graph C, what type of ecological fallacy bias is displayed?

Chapter 17 Qualitative research

Qualitative studies

A. Snowball sampling.
B. Maximum variation sampling.
C. Reliability.
D. Participant observation.
E. Negative sampling.
F. Focus group.
G. In-depth interview.
H. Reflexivity.
I. Transferability.
J. Quota sampling.

For each of the following definitions/statements, choose the most likely corresponding option from the list given above. Each answer can be used once, more than once or not at all.

1. Collecting data on naturally occurring behaviours of participants in their usual setting.
2. Using study participants as informants to identify other people who could potentially participate in the study.
3. Searching for unusual or atypical cases.
4. During the design phase of the study, a decision is made on how many people with certain characteristics are to be included as study participants.

5. The researcher reflects on whether his or her values and attributes may have influenced (or biased) any stages of the study.

Chapter 19 Screening, diagnosis and prognosis

Screening

A. 8813.
B. 10,000.
C. 99.95%.
D. 8809.
E. 5%.
F. 11.2%.
G. 76.
H. 63.32%.
I. 6.40%.
J. 0.05%.

Mammography is a common imaging tool used as a first screen for breast cancer. Assume the sensitivity and specificity of mammography in the detection of breast cancer are 95% and 88.8%, respectively. Assume the total number of people being imaged for breast cancer is 10,000 and that the prevalence of breast cancer in the population is 0.8%. The following 2 × 2 table can be used to summarize this information:

		Breast cancer		
		Yes	No	Total
Mammography	Positive	a	b	a + b
	Negative	c	d	c + d
	Total	a + c	b + d	10,000

For each question below, choose the most likely corresponding option from the list given above. Each answer can be used once, more than once or not at all.

1. What is the type 1 error of using mammography to detect breast cancer?
2. What is the type 2 error of using mammography to detect breast cancer?
3. What is the value of (c + d) from the table above?
4. What is the positive predictive value?
5. What is the negative predictive value?

Chapter 20 Statistical techniques

Calculating the P-value

A. Mann–Whitney U test.
B. Unpaired t-test.
C. McNemar's test.
D. One-sample t-test.

this process of randomization that makes RCTs the most rigorous method for determining a cause–effect relationship between an intervention and outcome, thus placing RCTs at the top of the hierarchy of evidence compared with the other study design options.

4. C. It would be sensible to use a case–control study design as:
   1. the outcome is rare (a case–control study design involves identifying all cases and controls at the start of the study). Apart from retrospective cohort studies, RCTs and prospective cohort studies are prospective in design and involve waiting for the outcome to occur.
   2. there may be a relatively long time lag between the exposure and outcome (no prospective follow-up is required in a case–control study design). Apart from retrospective cohort studies, RCTs and prospective cohort studies are prospective in design and involve waiting for the outcome to occur.
   3. little is known about the aetiology of the disease (a case–control study allows you to investigate whether a large number of exposures may be causing the disease). RCTs, prospective cohort studies and even retrospective cohort studies would not be helpful as little is known about what risk factors or exposures are causing the disease. Case reports sit low down on the hierarchy of evidence. A case report usually describes a single unique case or finding of interest. They are generally used to generate hypotheses, rather than test them.

5. D. Having demonstrated the effectiveness and safety profile of the new drug (using information from preclinical trials up to phase III trials), the drug can be subsequently licensed, marketed and made available for all patients. The main objective of phase IV trials is to gather information on:
   - how well the drug works in various populations.
   - the long-term risks and benefits of taking the drug.
   - the side effects and safety of the drug in larger populations.
   - whether the drug can be used in combination with other treatments (as in this example).

6. B. The five options all refer to different criteria from the Bradford Hill's criteria for causation between an exposure (gas emission) and outcome (respiratory disease).
   - Option A refers to 'reversibility': removing the exposure should reduce or prevent the disease outcome.
   - Option B refers to 'biological gradient (dose–response)': as in this example, there seems to be

a direct relationship between the level of exposure and the risk of disease.
   - Option C refers to 'consistency': numerous studies should be carried out before a statement can be made about the causal relationship between two variables.
   - Option D refers to 'biological plausibility': the apparent cause and effect must be plausible in the light of current knowledge.
   - Option E refers to 'temporal sequence': the exposure *must* always precede the outcome.

7. C. Let's work our way down the hierarchy of evidence (Chapter 2, Fig. 2.2).
   - A randomized controlled trial is not a good option as the research question does not involve a preventative measure or treatment.
   - A cohort study is a valid option; however, with a long time lag between exposure (head circumference at birth) and outcome (IQ), a retrospective study design is the most appropriate option.

8. D. A cross-sectional study is a form of observational study that involves collecting data from a target population at a single point in time. This methodology is particularly useful for assessing the true burden of a disease or the health needs of a population. Cross-sectional studies are therefore useful for planning the provision and allocation of health resources. Most government surveys conducted by the National Centre for Health Statistics are cross-sectional studies. Please refer to the respective Chapters for a discussion on the other study designs listed.

Chapter 11 Randomised controlled trials

1. B. Randomization ensures that those patient characteristics that may have an effect the outcome measure are distributed evenly between the groups. With this in mind, provided the trial is reasonably large, any observed differences between the study arms are due to differences in the treatment alone and not due to the effects of confounding factors (known or unknown) or selection bias.

2. C. This question requires you to calculate the number needed to treat (with the antidiabetic treatment) for harm (myocardial infarction):

$$= \frac{1}{|\text{Risk difference between two treatment groups}|}$$

$$= \frac{1}{(114 / 2500) - (61 / 2500)} = \frac{1}{0.0212} = 47$$

Therefore, 47 patients would need to be treated for 3 years (as this was the duration of the follow-up period in the study) with the new antidiabetic drug

303

to cause 1 extra myocardial infarction. Please refer to Chapter 12 for a further discussion on how to calculate the risk difference.

3. C. This study employs a factorial trial design, as two treatments (aspirin and beta-carotene) are evaluated *simultaneously* and compared with a control group (one control for each intervention) in the same trial. This type of randomized controlled trial is commonly used to evaluate interactions between treatments.
   - In a crossover trial, each subject acts as his or her own control, receiving all the treatments in a random sequence. In this particular study, patients would receive aspirin, beta-carotene or placebo in a random sequence.
   - In a parallel trial, each subject is randomly assigned to a group to receive only one of the treatments. In this particular study, patients would receive either aspirin, beta-carotene or placebo.
   - Cluster randomized trials involve groups of patients, clinics or communities, as opposed to individuals. These clusters are randomized to receive the intervention or a control. In this particular study, clusters of patients would receive either aspirin, beta-carotene or placebo.

   Preclinical trials involve using in vitro (test tube experiments) and in vivo (animal studies) techniques at a laboratory to obtain preliminary toxicity, efficacy and pharmacokinetic information on a new drug. This particular study is not a preclinical trial, but rather a clinical trial.

4. B. The answer to this question involves calculating the number needed to treat (NNT).

$$NNT = \frac{1}{\text{Risk difference between two treatment groups}}$$

The difference in outcome between the two groups, as denoted by the denominator of the formula above, is given as 25%.

$$NNT = \frac{100}{25} = 4$$

You therefore need to treat four patients with the new drug to prevent one hospital admission due to an acute exacerbation of asthma.

Chapter 12 Cohort studies

1. A. The biggest scientific issue in cohort studies is the loss of patients over time. Subjects, who are followed up until the outcome occurs or the study ends, may lose contact with the investigators, move out of the

area, die, etc. Loss-to-follow-up bias may be an issue if the reasons why patients are lost to follow-up are associated with *both the exposure and outcome*; for example, associated with exposed cases.
   - Patients are not recruited in cohort studies, which are observational in design.
   - There are no interventions in cohort studies as you are not intervening with usual practice.
   - Confounding is less of an issue than in case–control studies; therefore, this is not the biggest drawback of cohort studies.

   In general, cohort studies are less expensive than randomized controlled trials.

2. C. Healthy worker effect bias leads to an underestimation of the morbidity/mortality related to occupational exposures. In general, working individuals are healthier than the general population, which includes people who are unemployed because they are too sick to work.

Chapter 13 Case–control studies

1. C. The odds ratio indicates the increased (or decreased) odds of the disease being associated with the exposure of interest. The odds ratio can take any value between 0 and infinity. If the odds ratio is 0.87, the exposure of interest reduces the odds of disease by 13%. If the odds ratio was 1.87, the exposure of interest increases the odds of disease by 87 times.

2. D. Selecting up to four controls per case may improve the statistical power of the study to detect a difference between cases and controls. Including more than four controls per case does not generally increase the power of the study much further.

3. A. When the disease is not rare, the odds ratio can overestimate the risk ratio. The rest of the statements are correct.

4. E. The situation described is known as incidence–prevalence bias (also known as survival bias or Neyman bias), which is a type of ascertainment bias where the patients included in the study do not represent the cases arising in the target population. In incidence–prevalence bias, the sample of cases enrolled has a distorted frequency of exposure if the exposure itself (i.e., smoking) determines the prognosis (i.e., mortality) of the outcome (i.e., myocardial infarction).

It is also important to understand the difference between bias and confounding. In general, bias involves error in the measurement of a variable while confounding involves error in the interpretation of what may be an accurate measurement.

Chapter 14 Measures of disease occurrence and cross-sectional studies

1. B. The calculation is as follows:

$$\text{Incidence risk} = \frac{\text{Number of new cases of the disease in a given time period}}{\text{Population at risk (initially disease – free)}}$$

$$= \frac{300}{30000} = 0.01 = 1.0\%$$

2. D. The calculation is as follows:

$$\text{Incidence rate} = \frac{\text{Number of new cases of the disease}}{\text{Population at risk (initially disease – free)} \times \text{Time interval}}$$

$$= \frac{39}{4000 \times 3}\ 0.00325 \text{ cases per year}$$

$$= 325 \text{ cases per 100000 person - years}$$

3. E. It has been recognized that the decision for individuals in the study population to take part (or not take part) in a study is not random. A lower (not higher) socioeconomic status is associated with a low response rate.

Chapter 15 Ecological studies

1. E. Higher cholesterol levels are associated with a lower stroke mortality rate. However, at an individual level, there is a positive association between these two variables. This is referred to as a reversal of association. Please refer to Chapter 15, Fig. 15.1, and the accompanying text for a discussion on the other types of ecological fallacy.

Chapter 16 Case report and case series

1. D. Most case reports (and case series) cover one of six topics:
    1. Identifying and describing new diseases.
    2. Identifying rare or unique manifestations of known diseases.
    3. Audit, quality improvement and medical education.
    4. Understanding the pathogenesis of a disease.
    5. Detecting new drug side effects, both beneficial and adverse.
    6. Reporting unique therapeutic approaches.
    - Case studies do not involve satisfying a particular sample size, small or large.
    - Randomized controlled trials are most useful when determining a cause–effect relationship between an intervention and outcome.
    - Studies higher up in the hierarchy of evidence (systematic reviews (including meta-analyses), individual randomized controlled trials) are most useful for developing new practice guidelines.

2. D. Case series is a descriptive observational study that reports on data from a group of individuals who have a similar disease or condition (without a control group). Cases can be identified prospectively or retrospectively and can include either non-consecutive (a selection of cases) or consecutive individuals (all cases within a time frame) with the same disease or condition.

Chapter 17 Qualitative research

1. D. In purposive sampling, sample sizes are often determined by the saturation point. This is the point in data collection where interviewing new people will no longer bring additional insights to the research question. This theoretical saturation point can only be determined if data review and analysis are done in conjunction with data collection. This process is known as iteration, i.e. moving back and forth between sampling and analysis. Please refer to Chapter 17 for a full discussion on the two types of sampling methods mentioned (quota sampling and snowball sampling) and triangulation, which involves cross-verifying a research finding by using more than one research method.

2. B. Negative sampling (also known as deviant case sampling) involves searching for unusual or atypical cases of the research topic of interest. Please refer to Chapter 17 for a full discussion of the other types of sampling method options.

3. D. In qualitative research, the researcher should reflect on whether his or her values and attributes may have influenced (or biased) any stages of the study. This is often referred to as 'reflexivity'. Please refer to Chapter 17 for a full discussion of the remaining options.

Chapter 18 Confounding

1. B. The differences in BMI between the two groups would have occurred by chance (despite randomisation). BMI may be a confounding factor as there were differences in the BMI between the two treatment groups at the start of the trial and BMI may be related to blood pressure. As the trial is complete, confounding can be controlled for during the analysis phase of the study. It is important not to lose any information from the data when analysing the results, so excluding all patients in both groups with a BMI greater than 30 would be incorrect.

2. D. Effect modification is all about stratification and occurs when an exposure has a different effect on the outcome amongst different subgroups. In this example, the drug kavitab works better in reducing the risk of myocardial infarction in male than in female patients, compared to placebo. Gender is therefore an effect modifier.

Effect modification is different from confounding as instead of 'competing' with the exposure (the effect of kavitab) as an aetiological factor for the disease (myocardial infarction), the effect modifier (gender) identifies subpopulations (or subgroups) that are particularly susceptible to the exposure of interest. Effect modifiers are not on the causal pathway of the disease process.

If gender was a confounding factor, the stratum specific risk ratio of myocardial infarction amongst patients who took kavitab would be very similar in both male and female patients (but different from the crude estimate). Please refer to Chapter 15 for a discussion on effect modification in ecological studies.

Chapter 19 Screening, diagnosis and prognosis

1. D. Once you have extracted the true positive, false negative, true negative and false positive values from the question, the sensitivity, specificity, positive predictive value and negative predictive values can all be calculated.
    True positive = 567
    False negative = (1234 − 567) = 667
    True negative = 1145
    False positive = (1234 − 1145) = 89
    The calculations to help answer the question are as follow:
    The sensitivity of the new diagnostic test:

$$= \frac{\text{True positive}}{\text{True positive} + \text{False negative}}$$

$$= \frac{567}{567 + 667} = 45.9\%$$

The specificity of the new diagnostic test:

$$= \frac{\text{True negative}}{\text{True negative} + \text{False positive}}$$

$$= \frac{1145}{1145 + 89} = 92.8\%$$

The positive predictive value of the new diagnostic test:

$$= \frac{\text{True positive}}{\text{True positive} + \text{False positive}}$$

$$= \frac{567}{567 + 89} = 86.4\%$$

The negative predictive value of the new diagnostic test:

$$= \frac{\text{True negative}}{\text{True negative} + \text{False positive}}$$

$$= \frac{1145}{1145 + 667} = 63.2\%$$

2. D. The sensitivity and specificity describe the properties of the diagnostic test and are not dependent on the clinical sample (or target population). The sensitivity and specificity of a test are prevalence-independent. On the other hand, positive predictive values (and negative predictive values) are dependent on the population being studied (and therefore provide more clinically useful information). The positive predictive value increases (and the negative predictive value decreases) with a higher disease prevalence. Please refer to Chapter 8 for a discussion on P-values and confidence intervals.

3. B. The sensitivity and specificity of a test are prevalence-independent. In other words, assuming the performance of the test was rigorously investigated in the high prevalence population, the sensitivity and specificity should be the same in the low prevalence population. However, the predictive values are dependent on the prevalence of the disease in the population being studied. The only situation in which the predictive values are unaffected is when the sensitivity and specificity of the test are both 100%.
    The negative predictive value (NPV) can be written as:

$$\text{NPV} = \frac{\text{True negative}}{\text{True negative} + \text{False negative}}$$

As there are more people in the low prevalence population who will not have the disease, more people will have a negative test result and the negative predictive value will slightly increase.
The positive predictive value (PPV) can be written as:

$$\text{PPV} = \frac{\text{True positive}}{\text{True positive} + \text{False positive}}$$

As there are less people in the low prevalence population who have the disease, less people will have a positive test result and the positive predictive value will slightly decrease.

4. B.
    - Option A refers to spectrum bias.
    - Option B is correct: Partial verification bias (also known as work-up bias) occurs when the decision to perform the reference (gold standard) test on an individual is based on the results of the diagnostic study test.
    - Option C is incorrect: Partial verification bias may be avoided if the reference test is always performed prior to the study test.
    - Option D refers to differential verification bias.
    - Option E is incorrect: Partial verification bias cannot always be prevented. While it is possible to blind the investigator between the study test and reference test results, blinding may not

- Analysing the differences of numerical (specifically ratio) data (ESR level) across time categories. We are also told that the data follow a Gaussian distribution and that the variances (standard deviations) are constant between the groups.

4. B. The unpaired *t*-test is used to analyse the data, as we are:

- Comparing two independent (or unpaired) groups (medical students versus dental students).
- Analysing numerical (specifically interval) data (IQ), which follow a Gaussian distribution and have equal variances (standard deviations). IQ is an interval variable as there is no such thing as zero IQ. Furthermore, 120 IQ is not twice as intelligent as 60 IQ.

5. A. The Mann–Whitney U test (or the Wilcoxon two-sample signed rank test) is used to analyse the data, as we are:

- Comparing two independent (or unpaired) groups (lecture based versus problem based).
- Analysing numerical (specifically ratio) data (exam results) that do not follow a Gaussian distribution. The variances of the variable are also unequal between the two groups.

The 'test mark' variable is a ratio variable as:

- It includes a zero value; i.e., if all answers in the test are wrong.
- The questions are of equal difficulty. This means if someone has 60 correct answers, he has twice as many correct answers as someone with 30 correct answers (and he is twice as good in the module examined).

Chapter 21 Economic evaluation

Economic evaluation

1. D. Quality-adjusted life years (QALYs) for treatment B = $(12 \times 0.837) + (5 \times 0.516) = 12.62$ QALYs.

2. G. It is important to understand that the higher the EQ-5D health state score, the better the health. Intervention A is 'dominant' over intervention B, as the former is more effective and less expensive for each additional unit of health effect.

3. I.

$$ICER = \frac{\text{Cost of treatment A} - \text{Cost of no treatment}}{\text{Number of QALYs for treatment A} - \text{Number of QALYs for no treatment}}$$

$$= \frac{11000 - 0}{13.03 - 8.89} = £2657 \text{ per QALY}$$

4. F.

$$NMB = [(\text{Number of QALYs for treatment A} - \text{Number of QALYs for no treatment}) \times \lambda]$$
$$- (\text{Cost of treatment A} - \text{Cost of no treatment})$$

We are told that $\lambda = £30,000$.

$$NMB = [(13.03 - 8.89) \times 30000] - (11000 - 0)$$
$$= £113200$$

5. B. Utility measurements were combined with survival estimates to generate QALYs, which were used in a cost-utility analysis of competing healthcare interventions (treatment A versus treatment B).

Absolute risk reduction (ARR) Refer to definition for relative risk reduction (RRR).

Accuracy The closeness of the data to the true value.

Audit (or clinical audit) A technique used to examine clinical practice to determine the degree to which it meets agreed standards.

Bias (or systematic error) The phenomenon where a statistic is calculated in a way that makes the result systematically different from the true result. Bias can be divided into selection bias and measurement bias.

Blinding Patients and investigators (including those involved in recruitment and assessing the outcome) having no knowledge of treatment allocation.

The Bradford Hill criteria A group of nine principles that are used to establish epidemiological evidence of a causal relationship between a presumed cause (or exposure) and an observed effect (or outcome).

Case–control study A study in which patients with a certain condition (cases) are identified, along with similar patients without the condition (controls). Both groups are then assessed with the aim of identifying one or more factors which might account for the fact that cases have developed the condition and controls have not.

Case series A series of cases with a certain condition, with no controls.

Cluster randomized controlled trial A trial in which the intervention is randomly allocated to groups of patients (e.g., patients of one practice) rather than to individuals.

Cohort study A study in which patients who have been exposed to something (a possible cause of disease, or a drug) are compared to a similar group who were not exposed. It is usually prospective (subjects are followed up to see who develops the disease) but it can be retrospective (subjects' past histories are examined).

Confidence interval (CI), or confidence limits Describes a range of values. The 95% CI is the range within which there is a 95% chance that the true value for the population lies. The 95% confidence interval is roughly equal to two standard deviations about the mean.

Confounding Occurs when the association between an exposure and disease outcome is distorted by a third variable, which is known as a confounder. For instance, a study appears to show that standing in the street outside a public space causes lung cancer. Smoking is the confounder which makes smokers stand in the street and which causes lung cancer.

Cost–benefit analysis Measures the cost of an intervention and the benefit that ensues, both being measured in the same units (usually financial).

Cost–consequence analysis Measures the cost of the intervention and includes the nonhealth consequences.

Cost-effectiveness analysis Measures the costs and benefits of an intervention without describing them both in monetary terms.

Cost-effectiveness ratio (CER) The cost divided by the health outcome. The incremental cost-effectiveness ratio (ICER) is the difference in cost between two interventions divided by the difference in health effects.

Cost-minimization analysis Measures only the costs of alternative treatments. The benefits are assumed to be the same.

Cost-utility analysis Measures the benefits of an intervention in terms of personal preferences and describes the benefit in terms of what it costs to achieve a certain quality of gain, usually as the cost per quality-adjusted life year (QALY).

Cross-over study Analyses two or more groups, all of whom are exposed to all the interventions being tested, in turn.

Cross-sectional study An examination, at one point in time, of a sample, looking for the presence of variables (exposures, diseases, test results) that may be associated with each other.

Ecological studies Survey populations rather than individuals, looking for relationships between exposures and diseases. It can be at one point in time, or several points in time, comparing changes in the different populations.

Effectiveness Indicates whether the intervention works in practice.

Efficacy Indicates whether the intervention could work in practice if ideal conditions were met; for instance, that every patient completes the treatment.

Heterogeneity The word used in systematic reviews to describe the fact that different studies give different findings, suggesting that the results of each study are context specific. This means the results should not be combined.

Incidence The number of new cases of a certain disease occurring in a specified time.

Incidence rate The incidence risk in a specified unit of time; for example, 100 person-years.

Incidence risk The number of new cases divided by the number in the population at risk.

Intention to treat analysis The subjects of the study are analysed in the groups into which they were initially randomized. For instance, a subject randomized to treatment A is analysed in group A even if clinical necessity meant that the subject was changed to treatment B or left the trial all together.

Likelihood ratio Indicates how many times more likely it is that there will be a certain test result in a patient with the disease compared with a patient without the disease. The likelihood ratio for a positive result (LR+) is the proportion of people with the disease who have a positive test, divided by the proportion without the disease with a positive test. It is sensitivity divided by 1 – specificity; i.e., the true-positive rate over the false-positive rate. The likelihood ratio for a negative result (LR−) is the proportion of people with the disease who have a negative test divided by the proportion without the disease with a negative test. It is 1 – sensitivity divided by specificity; i.e., the false-negative rate over the true-negative rate.

Matching The technique of ensuring that, for every case, there are one or more controls who have the same characteristics; for example, sex, age, smoking status.

Mean The arithmetic mean, which is the sum of all the values divided by the number of values. The geometric mean is the mean calculated using log-transformed values.

Measurement bias Occurs when the information collected for the exposure and/or outcome variables is inaccurate. Measurement bias can be divided into random or nonrandom misclassification bias.

Meta-analysis A systematic review that summarizes the results of all eligible studies in a single figure.

Nonparametric statistics Does not assume that the data are normally distributed.

Nonrandom misclassification bias (also known as differential misclassification bias) Can lead to the effect of the exposure on the disease outcome being biased in either direction. This type of misclassification occurs only when the exposure measurement is related to the disease outcome status or vice versa.

Normal distribution, also called Gaussian distribution A distribution in which the different values are distributed symmetrically in a bell-shaped curve. Technically, it means that the mean = the median = the mode.

Number needed to treat for benefit (NNTB) The number who need to be treated for one of them to achieve the benefit in question. It is 1 divided by the risk difference.

Number needed to treat for harm (NNTH) The number who need to be treated for one of them to be harmed by the adverse effect in question. It is 1 divided by the risk difference, which is the percentage of subjects with that harm after the intervention minus the percentage of controls with that harm.

Odds The ratio of the probability of an event divided by the probability of no event. Where P = the probability, the odds are P divided by $1 – P$.

Odds ratio The odds of an event in cases divided by the odds of the event in controls.

Opportunity costs Are what is lost when resources are allocated to one intervention or service and not elsewhere.

Participant observation This is based on traditional ethnographic research whose objective is to understand perspectives held by study populations. Ethnographic research methods may include both observing people/processes and participating, to various degrees, in the day-to-day activities in the community setting.

Posttest odds The odds that the patient has the condition or disease after you know the result of the diagnostic test. It is the pretest odds times the likelihood ratio.

Posttest probability The likelihood that the patient has the condition or disease after you know the result of the diagnostic test. It is the posttest odds divided by 1 + posttest odds.

Power Refers to the ability of a study to detect a difference if there is one. If the study has sufficient power, then a negative result can be taken to mean that there is no effect from the intervention.

Precision The degree to which similar results are obtained on each testing. It is independent of accuracy.

Predictive values Estimates of how likely it is that a patient has, or does not have, the disease. The positive predictive value is the probability that the patient has the disease if the test is positive. The negative predictive value is the probability that the patient does not have the disease if the test is negative.

Pretest odds The odds that the patient has the condition or disease before you know the result of the diagnostic test. It is the pretest probability divided by 1 – pretest probability.

Pretest probability The likelihood that the patient has the condition or disease before you know the result of the diagnostic test.

Prevalence The proportion of people with the disorder in the population at the specified point in time.

Probability value (P) The probability that a result has arisen by chance. It is the same as the significance level. $P < 0.05$ means the probability that the result has arisen by chance is less than 5%.

Cohort studies *(Continued)*
  risk differences, 117–118, 118*t*, 222–223*t*
  risk ratios, 117, 118*t*, 222–223*t*
  subjects, 115
Commentaries, 77
Communication methods, teaching programme, 257
Comorbidities, RCT exclusion, 98*b*
Comparatior choice, RCTs, 98–99
Comparison, PICO, 5
Conclusions, case report writing, 158
Conference, curriculum vitae (CV) writing, 40
Confidence intervals, 63–64, 191, 222*t*
  independent proportions, difference between, 67–68
  means, 63–64
    difference between, 66–67
    reference range *vs.*, 64, 64*t*
    nonsignificant results, 72–73
      case study, 73
    paired means, difference between, 67
    power analysis *vs.*, 72
  for a proportion, 64–65
  risk ratios, 117
Conflict of interest, research study manuscript writing, 31
Confounding
  case–control studies, 130
  clinical appraisal, 216, 216*t*
  cohort studies, 118
  controlling for, 168–170
  cross-sectional studies, 143
  definition, 167, 167*f*
  disease associations, 167–168, 167*f*
  ecological studies, 152, 167
  example, 170–171
  exposure association, 167–168, 168*f*
  internal validity, 92
  observational studies, 167
  potential assessment, 167–168
  prognostic studies, 188
  RCTs, 102, 104
  result interpretation, 170
  result reporting, 170
Congenital abnormalities, case series example, 159
Consecutive sampling, clinical audit, 230
Consent, informed, 100
Consistency, Bradford–Hill criteria for causation, 93
Consolidated Standards of Reporting Trials (CONSORT), RCTs, 109, 110–112*t*, 112*f*
CONSORT (Consolidated Standards of Reporting Trials), RCTs, 109, 110–112*t*, 112*f*
Constrictive pericarditis, risk of, 129–130
Constructivist orientation, learning perspectives/theories, 251

Consultation, student in difficulty, 279–280
Contact information, curriculum vitae (CV) writing, 38
Contamination bias, RCTs, 103
Continuing professional development (CPD), curriculum vitae (CV) writing, 40, 247
Continuous probability distributions, 55–57
  normal (Gaussian) distribution. *(see* Normal (Gaussian) distribution)
  types, 56–57
Continuous variables, 46
Control
  case–control studies, 127
  PICO, 5
Control event rate, RCT results, 105
Control selection, case–control studies, 127
Core databases, 6, 6*b*
Correct summary measure choice, 59, 59*f*
Correlation coefficients, ecological studies, 150
Cost-benefit analysis, 210
Cost, economic evaluation, 200–201
Cost-effectiveness analysis, 208–209, 224*t*
  advantages, 210*b*
  disadvantages, 210*b*
  independent intervention, 208, 208–209*t*
  mutually exclusive interventions, 208–209, 209*t*
  questions and answers, 208–209
Cost-effectiveness ratio (CER), 224*t*
Cost-minimization analysis, economic evaluation, 201–202. *See also* Clinical equivalence
Cost-utility analysis, 224*t*
  advantages, 208
  disadvantages, 208
  economic evaluation, 202–208
Courses, curriculum vitae (CV) writing, 40
Cover letter, manuscript submission, 33–34
Critical appraisal, evidence identification, 9
Cross-over trials, RCTs, 107, 108*f*
Cross-sectional studies
  advantages, 145*b*
  analytical, 141
  bias, 143–145, 144*f*
    ascertainment bias, 144
    healthcare access bias, 144
    incidence-prevalence bias, 144, 145*f*
    measurement bias, 145
    migration bias, 145
    nonrandom misclassification bias, 145
    nonresponse bias, 144
    participation bias, 144
    random misclassification bias, 145
    selection bias, 143–145

Cross-sectional studies *(Continued)*
  causality, 143
  confounding, 143
  data collection, 140
  descriptive, 140–141
  disadvantages, 145, 145*b*
  key example, 146–147, 146*t*
  prevalence, 222–223*t*
  prevalence odds ratio, 222–223*t*
  prevalence ratio, 222–223*t*
  repeated, 141–142
  result interpretation, 142–143, 142*t*
    prevalence, 142
    prevalence odds ratio, 142–143, 143*t*
    prevalence ratio, 143, 143*t*
  study design, 140–142
Curriculum vitae (CV), 37
  common mistakes, 42
  style and formatting, 41*t*, 42
  writing
    audit and quality improvement, 40
    career aim, 38
    conferences, 40
    courses/continuing professional development, 40
    employment history, posts held, 39
    extra activities/personal interests, 41
    front sheet, 38
    gaps in employment, 39
    length, 37
    management and leadership experience, 40
    memberships, 38
    personal details and contact information, 38
    presentations, 39–40
    prizes and awards, 39
    professional registration, 38
    publications, 39
    qualifications, 38
    references, 41–42
    research experience, 39
    skills and experience, 41
    structure, 38

D

Data. *See also* Variables
  clinical audit, 231
  cross-sectional studies, 140
  quantitative (categorical) data, 46
  research design, 89–90
Data analysis/handling. *See also specific methods*
  clinical appraisal, 216
  correct summary measure choice, 59, 59*f*
  qualitative research, 163–164
  transformations, 57–58
Databases
  core, 6, 6*b*
  EMBASE, 6
  subject-specific, 6, 6*b*

Data collection methods, evaluation, 271
Definition of evidence-based medicine, 5
Demographic variables, mixed ecological studies, 151
Descriptive cross-sectional studies, 140–141
Design stage, controlling for confounding, 168–169
Detection bias
  case–control studies, 132–133
  RCTs, 104
Diagnosis
  definition, 173
  PICO, 5
  process of, 180–184
Diagnostic studies
  bias, 186–187
  clinical appraisal, 218–219
Diagnostic tests, 173, 177–178
  examples, 184–185
    equivocal pre-test probability/high prevalence, 185, 185t
    high pre-test probability/high prevalence, 185, 185t
    low pre-test probability/high prevalence, 184, 184t
  false negatives, 179
  false positives, 179
  frequency table, 178t
  likelihood ratios, 183, 183t
  negative predictive value, 178, 180
  performance evaluation, 178–180
  positive predictive value, 178, 180
  predictive values, 182
  pretest probability, 181
  screening tests vs., 173, 174t
  sensitivity, 178–179
  specificity, 178–179
  threshold, 178
  validity, 177–178
Diagnostic trials, 91
Dichotomous variables, 45
Differential verification bias, 186
Direction observation assessment methods, limitations of, 275
Direct observation of procedural skills (DOPS), 274
Discrete probability distributions, 57
Discrete variables, 46
Discussion
  case report writing, 158
  clinical appraisal, 216–217
  research study manuscript writing, 30
Discussion groups, small-group teaching, 260
Disease aspect, RCTs outcome, 99
Disease(s), confounding associations, 168
Disease-free survival, 188
Disease incidence, cohort studies, 222–223t
Disease occurrence. See Measures of disease occurrence

Disease odds, case–control studies, 222–223t
Disease odds ratio, case–control studies, 222–223t
Distributions
  binomial, 45
  frequency. (see Frequency distributions)
Documentation, search strategy, 8, 8b
Dose–response (biological grading), Bradford–Hill criteria for causation, 94
Dot plots, 51, 52f
Double distribution display, variables. See Variables

E

EBM. See Evidence-based medicine (EBM)
Ecological fallacy, 151f, 152–153
Ecological studies
  advantages, 154b
  confounding, 167
  data collection, 150
  disadvantages, 154b
  error sources, 152–154
    causality, 153
    confounders and modifiers, 153
    confounding by group, 152
    ecological fallacy, 151f, 152–153
    error modification by group, 153
    within-group bias, 152
  individual-level studies, 153–154
    design limitations, 153
    measurement limitation, 153–154
  inference, levels of, 149
  key example, 154
  measurement, levels of, 149
  mixed design, 150
  mixed studies, 151–152
  modifiers, 153
  result interpretation, 150–152
    correlation coefficients, 150
    regression analysis, 150
    scatter plots, 150, 151f
  study design, 149–150
  types, 149–150
Ecologic inferences, 149
Economical costs, 199
Economic aspects, RCTs outcome, 99
Economic evaluation, 224, 224t
  cost-benefit analysis. (see Cost-benefit analysis)
  cost-effectiveness analysis. (see Cost-effectiveness analysis)
  cost-minimization analysis, 201–202 (see also Clinical equivalence)
  costs, 200–201
  cost-utility analysis. (see Cost-utility analysis)
  economic questions, 200–201
  health utilities. (see Health utilities)
  net monetary benefit, 207

Economic evaluation (Continued)
  quality-adjusted life years. (see Quality-adjusted life years (QALYs))
  sensitivity analysis, 210–212
  study design, 200–201
Economics, health. See Health economics
Edited book, chapters, 31–32
Effectiveness and Efficiency: Random Reflections on Health Service (Cochrane), 77
Effectiveness, RCT results, 105
Effective teaching materials, 268–269
  educational impact, feedback, 269
  evidence-based medicine and teaching, 268–269
Effective teaching session, 253
  Bloom's taxonomy, 254–255, 255–256t
  lesson plan component, 254t
  setting objectives, 253–255
  SMART objectives, 253–254
Effect size, statistical power, 74
Efficacy, RCT results, 105
Efficiency, health economics, 199
EMBASE database, 6
Employment history, curriculum vitae (CV) writing, 39
Environmental measures, ecological studies, 149
EQ-5D method, health utilities, 205, 207t
Equivalence trials
  clinical equivalence, 202, 202f
  RCTs, 108
Error bars, 68
Error modification by group, ecological studies, 153
Errors
  type I, 70–71
  type II, 71
Estimate combination, meta-analyses, 78
Ethical issues
  clinical appraisal, 215
  RCTs, 99–100
Ethnographic research methods, 162
Evaluation, 271–272
  analysis and action, 272
  completing, 271–272
  data collection methods, 271
  evaluation focus, 271
  focus, 271
  goals of, 271
  peer evaluation, 272
  self-evaluation, 272
  students, 272
Evidence
  bias in meta-analyses, 82
  gap identification, 15–16, 15t
  hierarchy of. (see Hierarchy of evidence)
Evidence-based medicine (EBM)
  definition of, 5
  teaching materials, 268–269
Evidence dissemination, bias in meta-analyses, 82

Evidence identification
  critical appraisal, 9
  hierarchy of evidence, 9, 9*f*
  information sources, 6
  search strategy, 6
Evidence synthesis, 78
Exclusion bias, case–control studies, 132
Exclusion criteria
  case series, 158
  RCTs, 97–98
Explicit criteria, clinical audit,
    229, 232*t*
Exposure, confounding association,
    167–168, 168*f*
Exposure odds, case–control studies,
    222–223*t*
Exposure odds ratio, case–control studies,
    222–223*t*
Exposure status measurement, case–
    control studies, 127–128
Exposure suspicion bias, cohort studies, 121
External validity
  clinical appraisal, 215
  evidence critical appraisal, 9
  RCTs, 97–98
Extra activities/personal interests,
    curriculum vitae (CV)
    writing, 41

F

Factorial trials, RCTs, 108, 108*t*
Fagan nomogram, 183, 183*f*
False negatives (FN), 223*t*
  diagnostic tests, 178–179
False positives (FP), 223*t*
  diagnostic tests, 178–179
F-distribution, 57
Feedback, 275–276
  process of, 275
  provider, 276
  receiver, 276
Financial costs, 199
Fisher's exact test, 193
Five-year survival, mortality, 188
Fixed-effects meta-analysis, pooled
    estimate calculations, 79
FN. *See* False negatives (FN)
Focus groups, qualitative research, 162
Follow-up
  cohort studies, 116
  prognostic studies, 188
  student in difficulty, 280, 280*t*
FP. *See* False positives (FP)
Free-text searches, 7
Frequency distributions, 46*t*, 47, 221, 221*t*
  arithmetic mean, 52
  bar charts, 47, 48*f*
  central tendency, 51–53
  histograms, 47–49, 49*t*, 50*f*
  pie charts, 47, 48*f*
  variability, 53–54

Front sheet, curriculum vitae (CV)
    writing, 38
Funnel plots, 82
  asymmetry, 82–83

G

Gaussian distribution. *See* Normal
    (Gaussian) distribution
General Medical Council (GMC), 3, 37, 280
Geographical studies, 149
Geometric means, 57, 58*t*
Global measures, ecological studies, 149
Good Medical Practice, 3
Group effect modification, 153
Group learning, teaching methods, 259

H

Handouts, large groups/lecturing, 264
Healthcare access bias
  case–control studies, 133
  cohort studies, 120
  cross-sectional studies, 144
Healthcare professionals, 3–4
Health economics
  definition, 199–200
  efficiency, 199
  evaluation. (*see* Economic evaluation)
  opportunity costs, 199–200
Health utilities, 202–205
  direct measurement, 203
  indirect measurements, 204–205
  public *vs.* patients, 204, 205*t*
  standard gamble, 204
  time trade-off, 203–204
  visual analogue scale, 203–204
Health worker effect bias, 120
Heterogeneity
  degree estimation, 79
  meta-analyses, 78–79
  options for, 79–80
  sources of, 79
  tests for, 78–79
Hierarchy of evidence, 9, 9*f*
  choice of research design, 94–96
Histograms, frequency distributions,
    47–49, 49*t*, 50*f*
Hospital admission rate bias, 131–132
Humanist orientation, learning
    perspectives/theories, 248–250
Hypothesis, null. *See* Null hypothesis
Hypothesis testing, 61
  alternative. (*see* Alternative hypothesis)
  null hypothesis, 61, 69
  sample choice, 61
  statistical, 69

I

ICER (incremental cost-effectiveness
    ratio), 205, 224*t*

Illustrations, creativity, 25
Implicit criteria, clinical audit, 231, 232*t*
Incidence, 137–139. *See also* Measures of
    disease occurrence
  prevalence *vs.*, 139–140, 140*f*
Incidence–prevalence bias
  case–control studies, 133
  cross-sectional studies, 144, 145*f*
Incidence rates, 137–139
  mixed ecological studies, 151
Inclusion bias, case–control studies, 132
Inclusion criteria
  case series, 158
  RCTs, 97–98
Incremental cost-effectiveness ratio
    (ICER), 205, 224*t*
Independent events, rules of probability, 55
Independent intervention, cost-
    effectiveness analysis, 208,
    208–209*t*
Independent proportions, difference
    between, 67–68
In-depth interviews, 162
Information. *See also specific sources*
  evidence identification, 6
  informed consent, 100
Informed consent, RCTs, 100
Inspiration, clinical audit, 228–229
Institute for Healthcare Improvement, 235
Instructional teaching strategies, 255,
    255–256*t*
Integrated academic training pathways,
    13, 13*f*
Intention to treat (ITT) analysis, RCT
    results, 105
Interests, research project supervisor, 16
Interim analysis, RCT results, 105
Internal validity
  bias, 92
  causality, 92
  clinical appraisal, 215
  confounding, 92
  evidence critical appraisal, 9
International Medical Education (IIME),
    247
Interquartile range, frequency
    distributions, 54
Interval variables, 45–46
Interventional studies, 90. *See also specific
    trials*
  choice of, 97
  validity, 90
Intervention bias, allocation of, 103
Intervention event rates, RCT
    results, 105
Interventions
  PICO, 5
  student in difficulty, 280, 280*t*
Interviewer bias
  cohort studies, 121–122
  RCTs, 104
Interviews, in-depth, 162

Introductions
    case report writing, 157
    research study manuscript writing, 29
ITT (intention to treat) analysis, RCT
    results, 105

J

Joint Royal Colleges of Physicians Training
    Board, 274
Journal articles, references, 31
Journal selection, manuscript submission,
    32–33

L

Large groups/lecturing, teaching methods,
    263–265, 264b
Large samples, 63, 65
Leadership experience, curriculum vitae
    (CV) writing, 40
Lead-time bias, screening programmes,
    175, 176f
Learning theory
    behaviourist orientation, 247–248
    cognitivist orientation, 248
    constructivist orientation, 251
    humanist orientation, 248–250
    medical education, 247–251
    social learning orientation, 250–251
Lecture activities, large groups/lecturing,
    264–265
Lecture content, large groups/lecturing, 264
Lecture/presentation, references, 32
Length time bias, screening programmes,
    175, 176f
Lesson plan component, 254t
Levels of evidence, 15, 15t
Likelihood ratios
    diagnostic tests, 183, 183t
    posttest probability, 182–183
Literature reviews, 77
Logarithmic transformations, 57–58
Loss-to-follow-up bias
    cohort studies, 119–120
    diagnostic studies, 187
    RCTs, 104

M

Management, curriculum vitae (CV)
    writing, 40
Manuscript submission, 32–34
    cover letter, 33–34
    instructions for authors, 33
    journal selection, 32–33
    presubmission checklist, 34
Maslow's hierarchy of needs, 248, 250f
Matching
    case–control studies, 127
    controlling for confounding, 169
Mathematical modelling, 170

Maximum variation sampling, qualitative
    research, 163
Means
    arithmetic. (*see* Arithmetic mean)
    difference between, confidence
      intervals, 66–67
    geometric, 57, 58t
Measurement bias
    case–control studies, 133–134
    clinical appraisal, 217t
    cohort studies, 120–122
    cross-sectional studies, 145
    RCTs, 104
Measures of disease occurrence, 137–140
    incidence, 137
    incidence rate, 137
    prevalence, 137
Median, frequency distributions, 53, 53f
Median survival, mortality, 188
Medical education, 247
    behaviourist orientation, 247–248
    cognitivist orientation, 248
    constructivist orientation, 251
    humanist orientation, 248–250
    learning perspectives/theories, 247–251
    medical education, 247–251
    optimizing learning, 251, 251t
    social learning orientation, 250–251
    technology in, 267
MEDLINE database, 6
Memberships, curriculum vitae (CV)
    writing, 38
Meta-analyses, 78–81. *See also* Systematic
    reviews
    bias, 82
      evidence dissemination, 82
      evidence production, 82
    clinical appraisal, 217–218
    estimate combination, 78
    evaluation, 81–83
    example, 84–85
    fixed effect *vs.* random effect, 80
    heterogeneity, 78–79
    necessity for, 78
    pooled estimate calculations, 79
    presentation, 81
    publication bias, 82–83
    random effect, 79–80
    result interpretation, 81–82
    sensitivity analysis, 81
    subgroup analysis, 80
Methods, research study manuscript
    writing, 29–30
Migration bias
    case–control studies, 133
    cross-sectional studies, 145
Mini-clinical evaluation exercise
    (mini-CEX), workplace-based
    assessment, 274
Minimisation randomisation, RCTs, 101
Mode, frequency distributions, 52–53, 53f
Modernizing Medical Careers (MMC), 13

Modifiers, ecological studies, 153
Morbidity, 188
Mortality, 188
    definition, 139b
Multinomial variables, 45
Multiple myeloma, case report example,
    159
Multiple-source feedback (MSF),
    workplace-based assessment, 275
Multiway sensitivity analysis, economic
    evaluation, 211
Mutually exclusive events, rules of
    probability, 55
Mutually exclusive interventions, cost-
    effectiveness analysis, 208–209,
    209t

N

Narrative reviews, 77
Negative likelihood ratio, 223t
Negatively skewed probability
    distributions, 57
Negative predictive value (NPV), 223t
    diagnostic process, 180
    diagnostic tests, 178, 180
    positive predictive value *vs.*, 180
Negative sampling, qualitative research,
    163
Net monetary benefit (NMB), 223t
    economic evaluation, 207
NMB. *See* Net monetary benefit (NMB)
NNTB. *See* Numbers needed to treat to
    benefit (NNTB)
NNTH. *See* Numbers needed to treat to
    harm (NNTH)
Nominal variables, 45
Non-fatal incidents, morbidity, 188
Non-Gaussian distributions, Gaussian
    distribution *vs.*, 191–192
Noninferiority trials, 202
    clinical equivalence, 202, 203f
Non-parametric tests, 191–192
    null hypothesis, 191
Non-random misclassification bias
    case–control studies, 134
    cohort studies, 121–122
    cross-sectional studies, 145
    RCTs, 104
Non-research projects, types of, 14–15, 14t
Non-response bias
    case–control studies, 132
    cohort studies, 120
    cross-sectional studies, 144
Normal (Gaussian) distribution, 55–56
    non-Gaussian distributions *vs.*, 191–192
    reference range, 56
    standard normal distribution, 56
NPV. *See* Negative predictive value (NPV)
Null hypothesis, 61
    equivalence trials, 202
    non-inferiority trials, 202

Variables *(Continued)*
  nominal, 45
  ordinal, 45
  single distribution display, 47–49, 47t.
    See also specific methods
  types of, 191
Verification bias, 186
Video, creativity, 25, 25t
Visual analogue scale, health utilities,
  203–204

W

Ward teaching, clinical environment
  teaching, 263
Websites, references, 32
Within-group bias, 152
Working environment, research project
  supervisor, 16
Workplace-based assessment, 274–275
  assessor training, 275
  case-based discussion, 274–275
  direction observation assessment
    methods, limitations of, 275
  direct observation of procedural skills,
    274
  mini-clinical evaluation exercise, 274
  multiple-source feedback, 275
Work-up bias, 186
Written assessment, 272, 273t